I0108901

Seven Nights with Ayahuasca

A graphic account of heaven and hell, and the bizarre infinity in between

By Nicholas Floyd

Also by Nicholas Floyd

You Can't Spell Tokyo Without K.O.
A photo-essay dissecting the Japanese epidemic
of passing out in public

Copyright © 2015 Nicholas Floyd

This book may be freely reproduced (in part or in whole) for personal and noncommercial use, under the following two conditions:

(1) the book's text is unmodified
(2) the book's full title and author's name are conspicuous

Where purchasing a copy is not viable, sharing a copy is highly encouraged.

No part of this book may be reproduced for commercial gain of any sort, whether directly (via sales) or indirectly (via peripheral advertising, etc.), without permission of the copyright holder, with the exception of reviewers, who may quote brief passages in reviews.

ISBN: 978-0-9961732-0-9
Third revision (April, 2023)

Issued also in digital format.

Cover art by Misprint.
www.misprint.com.au

Cover design by Jennifer Quinlan.
www.historicaleditorial.com

To everyone I've ever wronged.

Table of Contents

Preface

This is a work of nonfiction. In order to convey the events accurately — in the same vivid and explicit manner that they were experienced — this book contains extremely graphic sexual descriptions. This book also contains graphic descriptions of gore and unpleasant bodily functions such as vomiting and diarrhea. Reader discretion is strongly advised.

. . .

Passages written in *italic lettering* denote immersive visions and other psychedelic effects induced by Ayahuasca. The details described therein should not be interpreted as hypotheses or claims about the objective nature of the universe.

. . .

While many Ayahuasca visions convey clear meaning or psychological origin, others do not. This book is intentionally devoid of speculative analysis, and the reader is encouraged to draw their own conclusions about the possible meaning, if any, of such visions.

Prologue

Before drinking Ayahuasca, it's as if I had lived my life confined in a dark, windowless room locked from the inside. I spent most of my life peering out of the door's narrow keyhole — my normal waking consciousness — which revealed only the sliver of the world right in front of me. From my tiptoes I could peer out of the fisheye lens of the peephole — my dream consciousness — which offered a wider view, but one that was warped, blurry, and difficult to comprehend. My limited perception of the world reinforced my natural assumption that it centered around me.

Thin beams of light seeped into the room from the outside through the keyhole, illuminating tiny patches of my body and offering minor clues as to who I might be, but I remained largely unaware of myself and the world around me. Occasionally I stepped on something sharp or bumped into something painful, but the darkness concealed what exactly had hurt me, and the true extent of my injuries.

If I had learned psychological lock picking via meditation, perhaps I could have escaped my dark confinement without the need for a key. But it turned out that Ayahuasca — one of the keys that could unlock the door — happened to be sitting within reach the whole time. I simply needed to find it, and then gather the courage to use it. Once I finally stepped out of the darkness to behold the world, its enormity and breathtaking beauty astonished me. Yet at the same time, a hideous abomination repulsed me. Right outside stood a mirror in which I saw myself fully illuminated for the first time: the sharp thorns of regret lodged in my flesh, the jagged splinters of past trauma buried in my heels, the irritating rashes of needless worry upon my face, and my frightening scowl of selfishness. Understanding the causes of my pain was the first step in

2

alleviating it, and seeing my ugly side was the first step in addressing it.

That's where the analogy ends though, because the experience of drinking Ayahuasca proved far more difficult than simply turning a key and looking into a mirror. When I was in the jungle wallowing in the brutal pangs of Ayahuasca intoxication, ravaged by sharp cramping and a turbulent whirlwind of emotions, at times it felt impossible to endure. I grimaced and groaned and gritted my teeth. Several times I wept, and I silently begged for it all to stop. The terrifying realism of the immersive visions temporarily convinced me that I had lost my sanity, and that I would never be myself again.

But my fellow participants in the jungle corroborated my conclusion that despite the painful and arduous tribulations, emerging on the other side of the experience can be euphoric and profound, and though it won't necessarily change you as a person, it probably will change your understanding of yourself, and your outlook on life. You might find that your ego has been whittled down, and that you no longer see yourself as the center of the universe. You might be shocked by the rejuvenation of shedding the excess emotional weight that you had carried, the true gravity of which might have eluded you with its slow and gradual build over the years.

And like any truly harrowing experience, you shouldn't be surprised or ashamed to find that you shat yourself.

Departure from Civilization

Under different life circumstances, perhaps I would have been hesitant about spending ten days with two dozen strangers in the depths of the Amazon rainforest, cut off from civilization, sleeping in a thatched roof hut with no electricity and no running water, ingesting a shaman's magic potion of epic potency. However, I had spent the last four years of my life slogging through the hell of Tokyo's corporate world — bludgeoned black and blue by the endless stresses of work, routinely assaulted by the constant commotion of life in a megalopolis, severed from nature aside from the occasional fleeting glimpse of the setting sun viewed from an office skyscraper — all of which culminated in my intense yearning for the quiet isolation of the remote jungle, for a reconnection with nature, and for a profound mental reset. My life needed to change course, but I didn't know which direction, and I didn't realize the extent to which civilization had already taken a toll on me. I was unknowingly mutating into a crotchety young man viewing the world through a lens tainted with misanthropy and bitterness, and my entire journey to the jungle only soured me further.

If it had been my first time with intercontinental travel, perhaps I would have dreaded the twenty-four hours required to get to Iquitos, Peru, especially considering that after Iquitos I still had another three hours to go, first by bus, then by boat, then by foot. But a decade-plus of back and forth between continents had already prepared me to endure the vortex of intercontinental travel — that blurry and surreal purgatory inhabited by caffeine-fueled specters.

Spending those twenty-four hours in a sleepless daze might have felt like a squandered opportunity for last-minute mental preparation, except that I had already spent over a year immersing myself in countless books, documentaries, articles, podcasts, and first-person testimonials regarding Ayahuasca and its psychoactive component, DMT. A constant, low-level anxiety coursed through me, but I felt as prepared as possible, and I knew that further preparation would be impractical anyway, in the hazy pseudo-consciousness and mild delirium that come standard with intercontinental travel.

After landing in Lima, I fumbled my way through the haze of one more layover and one more flight, both indistinguishable from my previous layovers and flights, except that most of caffeine-fueled specters now spoke Spanish. My infantile grasp of the language allowed me to easily tune it out, offering a thin barrier of protection between me and the constant commotion of civilization from which I fled. But that barrier dissipated as soon as I set foot outside the airport and into the unfamiliar streets of Iquitos.

The city's most prominent feature struck me first: the infestation of motorized tricycle taxis, whose air pollution and noise pollution walloped me with a one-two punch. The stinging smog scratched at my lungs, and my burning eyes corroborated that indeed the air seemed toxic.

The city's second-most prominent feature struck me next: the legions of disheveled stray dogs that hobbled about the streets, afflicted with various ailments. Some appeared to have rabies, with long beards of foamy saliva hanging from their jaws. Some appeared to have leprosy, with patchy chunks of fur missing. Unprotected from the relentless tropical sun, their bald patches glowed from chronic sunburn, a dark hue of pinkish red like cured meats. Some of the strays suffered from fresh wounds yet to heal, while others suffered from old sores oozing with pus.

I raced to my hotel and checked in with the hospitable staff who then showed me to my room, which they had pre-chilled to the frigid temperature of a walk-in refrigerator. The rattling air conditioner appeared several decades old, faded to the dirty yellow hue of a chain smoker's fingernails, and it struggled as it coughed out what smelled like moldy Freon. I thanked and tipped the hotel staff, shut the door behind them, immediately laid the air conditioner to rest, and then set out to procure jungle supplies before sundown, in preparation for the next day's hike to the retreat grounds.

In accordance with the retreat's guidelines, for the past two weeks I had abstained from all sexual activity, including masturbation. When I had read the retreat's brochure several weeks prior, their policy of mandatory sexual abstinence struck me as dubious, especially given the track record of organizations that have imposed sexual abstinence, and the tendency of those policies to backfire. The retreat attempted to justify their abstinence policy by claiming that it allowed for mental concentration and devotion of our full attention, but I knew from past experience that harboring inside of me a raging pressure cooker of repressed natural instinct would not be conducive to mental concentration. The policy didn't present to me any challenges of willpower, but it concerned me for reasons of efficacy and practicality.

Nonetheless, I had given them the benefit of the doubt, resolving myself to temporary abstinence, rationalizing that thousands of years of shamanic tradition probably produced more wisdom than my twenty-something years of masturbating.

As I trekked through the streets of Iquitos with an unwanted accumulation of testosterone within me, my heightened senses picked up the voluptuous silhouette of a woman in the distance. From afar I couldn't make out her facial features or skin tone, but her ludicrous waist-to-hip ratio, bountiful chest, and pronounced backside suggested that she was gifted with the finest of Latin American genetics. I knew that the retreat's abstinence policy, the insurmountable language barrier, and my own moral convictions precluded any chance of a sexual encounter, but an ambient Siren's song drifted into my ears and beckoned me to come hither, just to say hello with a quick glance.

The wildly proportioned female silhouette drew closer into view, revealing her unexpected identity: a faceless mannequin, positioned outside a clothing store. At first I assumed that no mannequin could possibly have such pronounced curvature, and that the repressed sexual energy polluting my mind must be distorting my perception, but drawing closer revealed that the mannequin did indeed wield the outrageous physical features of an adult entertainer.

The bustling noise and stinging stench of the Iquitos streets faded out, and everything in the periphery blurred away as I stared with acute tunnel vision at the inanimate temptress. Without my consent, a rogue surge of blood flowed through my neglected genitals and threatened to engorge me, but I chose not to heed the warning, under the assumption that my own shame would be sufficient deterrent to prevent being aroused by a faceless mannequin. That quickly proved untrue, forcing me to avert my eyes and scurry off with one hand in my pocket, attempting to contain my embarrassing semi-engorgement.

My mind raced to think of unsexy thoughts, and a commotion in a nearby alley offered a much needed distraction. An unruly mob of ravenous vultures, dozens in number, thrashed about in piles of rotting garbage, their beaks tearing at the rubbish as they squawked and jockeyed for position. They stabbed and lashed at each other, establishing a brutal pecking order, with the largest, most ferocious of them indulging in the filthy spoils. Amidst the heinous screeching and cawing, from off in the distance the hoarse shouting of a decrepit old man echoed through the streets as he expended the last of his strength, crying forth exasperated but zealous tirades in Spanish. Though unintelligible to me, his rasping sounded like a soothsayer's grim premonitions of the end times, which seemed to be unfolding in the alley before my eyes.

The distraction allowed my semi-engorged member to deflate, and I stood in a dumbfounded stupor, trying to make sense of the scene. At the same time, a flock of adolescent street hawkers picked up the scent of my gringo trail, swooping in and encircling me. Before I could snap out of my stupor, I found myself center stage in a pop-up bazaar of small children, each touting their various crafts and jewelry at exorbitant prices set specifically for tourists. Nearly a dozen handfuls of goods continually thrust toward my face amidst shouts of "authentic" and "handmade", and I noticed that many of the hawkers touted suspiciously similar items — thread for thread and bead for bead — which I assumed were mass-produced on a factory assembly line.

An aggressive tugging pulled down the side of my shirt, and when I made the mistake of looking over, a young boy locked eyes with me, thrust a handful of bracelets in my face, and repeatedly shouted.

"For me schooool! For me schooool!"

If the sale would have truly financed his education, perhaps the inauthenticity and preposterous asking price would not have fazed me, but his brand-name sneakers and New York Knicks basketball cap, both spotless and new, cast serious doubt upon the legitimacy of his claims. The sale likely would have funded the matching jersey to go with his cap, so I declined his offer, which he repeated another eight times while relentlessly tugging at my shirt.

A steep language barrier stood between us, so I attempted to ward off the throng of hawkers by gesturing the universal empty pocket motion for "I'm broke". One of the boys then gestured an offer to buy my shorts — the pair that I currently wore — under the false impression that they were name brand or had any value.

8

When it became obvious to them that I was an unprofitable venture, the throng disbanded in search of other, more lucrative gringos. I likewise hurried off, in a rush to get off the streets after purchasing the one thing that I needed: rubber boots in preparation for the next day's muddy jungle hike. I snatched up the first pair in sight, without even trying them on, then darted back to my hotel and relished in my first real rest in thirty-six hours.

At sunrise I convulsed awake to what sounded like clanging pots and pans. With foggy eyes I turned my head to see the room's exposed pipes clanking and trembling, perhaps because of faulty plumbing, perhaps because someone down below kept banging them with a hammer. Exhaustion and sleep deprivation still overwhelmed me, so I waited in hopes that the racket would cease, but when the intensity only increased, I conceded defeat and rose from bed.

Inside the bathroom I discarded my shirt and dropped my drawers, emptying what would potentially be my last solid bowel movement for the next ten days, into what would certainly be the last Western toilet that I would see for the next ten days. My follow-up shower washed away some of my grogginess and jetlag, refreshing me enough to pack my one lone bag and then head toward the hotel lobby, the retreat's scheduled pick-up point.

Aside from carrying far less luggage than most, I fit right in with the lobby's congregation of apprehensive and bumbling foreigners. We made our unceremonious acquaintances with each other, initiated by self-introductions based on the loose assumption that, as fellow confused-looking foreigners with jungle gear, we must be headed to the same place. Some folks appeared well versed in bold international adventures, showing no signs of anxiety. Other folks did not appear well versed in adventure of any kind, fidgeting about while checking and rechecking their numerous bags. But to my surprise the group seemed devoid of the thrill-seeking and pretentious neo-hippies that, in my misanthropic state of mind, I had presumed would inundate the retreat. Rather, a variety of cultural backgrounds comprised the eclectic group, which appeared to span an age range of at least four decades, and generally everyone made a good first impression.

Outside of the hotel, our ride — a dilapidated, long-retired school bus from Korea — pulled up amidst a thick cloud of dirt and exhaust, trailed by a flock of clamoring street hawkers. They thrust their merchandise and shouted their "discount" prices at us as we filed into the bus, but most of the hawkers stood dejected without a sale as our ramshackle bus's wheezing engine summoned the energy to depart.

Along our way to the boat port, the musty odor of old vinyl seats mixed with an already pungent cloud of body odor, helping to dilute the stinging air pollution of the Iquitos streets. Throughout the forty-five-minute journey, we hit countless devastating potholes and craters, but our dilapidated Korean school bus managed to hold together and safely deliver us to a run-down port on the Nanay River, a tributary of the Amazon River.

Unattended children and stray dogs scampered around as rifle-wielding commercial boat crews loaded their cargo of thatches. A trio of children swam and frolicked in the shallow waters nearby, blissfully indifferent to the danger of snakes and alligators and piranhas, and equally indifferent to the thick, bubbly film of beige goo that coated the polluted riverbanks like a floating blanket of mold. The children smiled and giggled as they pointed at our motley crew of predominantly pasty white, camera-toting foreigners.

We loaded our cargo onto a boat far less dilapidated and far less Korean than the bus we rode in on. As we filed onboard one by one, most of us advertised through a wobbly lack of balance that it was likely our first time boarding a jungle boat via a rickety, lopsided plank.

The last passenger boarded, the land crew shoved us off, and I bid farewell to the port's polluted riverbanks as we pulled away. We gathered speed downstream, and a refreshing breeze of crisp jungle air streamed across my face as I bid farewell to the stinging airborne toxins of Iquitos. The last signs of civilization faded out of sight beyond the river bend behind us, and so too faded from my mind the noise and commotion of everyday life, the misery of the corporate world, the dizzying vortex of intercontinental air travel, and the chronic malcontent that had plagued me. Speeding along the calm waters toward the start of my true journey, I felt something that I almost didn't recognize: a glimmer of optimism.

Arrival and Orientation

After thirty minutes of high-speed getaway on the Nanay River, our captain cut the boat's engine and veered into a narrow inlet. We coasted in silence, and no one dared to utter a sound as we listened with reverence to the melodic chirping and singing of birds, the bass and baritone croaking of frogs, the buzzing hum and percussion clicks of insects, and the soft stirring of leaves blowing in the wind, all combined into a pacifying jungle symphony. Upon the massively elevated water levels of the Amazonian rainy season, we cruised above underwater treetops, their leaves and branches rustling as they caressed the underside of our boat, and our captain navigated through the inlet's narrow twists and turns. The enormity and complexity of the jungle humbled me, and simply being there vanquished any thoughts of the tribulations thus far.

Our captain docked next to a steep embankment where we unloaded and began our forty-five-minute hike even deeper into the flooded jungle terrain. The rubber boots that I had purchased in haste the day prior turned out to be a full size too large, and with each slippery, muddy step, my feet grated against the rough rubber confines. Halfway through the hike a thick layer of chafed flesh peeled from the ball of my left foot, tearing further and further with each step. I considered forgoing the rubber boots altogether and reverting to my tennis shoes, but I nixed that idea at the thought of ruining my only pair of shoes, and at the more unpleasant thought of having to go shopping for a replacement pair, in Iquitos or elsewhere.

We arrived sweaty and exhausted at the entrance to the retreat grounds, where five shamans short of stature stood wearing traditional Shipibo garb. Each shaman greeted us with an enthusiastic smile and hug, unfazed by our shirts sopping with sweat. Our massive difference in height required me to fully bend over at the waist to exchange hugs with one of the shortest shamans. She tugged at my long-sleeved pajama shirt and matching pajama pants, unable to contain her lighthearted laughter, chuckling to the other four in their native tongue what I presumed to mean, "Didn't anyone tell this white boy it's hot in the jungle!?"

Though it looked foolish, I deliberately chose long pajamas for two main benefits. First, the thin and well-ventilated fabric protected me from mosquitoes while staying cool. Second, the disposable pajamas offered peace of mind because I had purchased them for a negligible price from a thrift store, with the expectation of ruining them by vomiting on myself or soiling myself or both.

My fellow participants and I stood around waiting for the last few stragglers to catch up, and several of us looked each other up and down, wide-eyed in disbelief, mutually toiling over the absurdity of each other's clothing choices. In stark contrast to my armor of long pajamas tucked into tube socks and rubber boots, some folks wore a minimal attire of tank top, sandals, and shorts. Several women wore shorts that exposed the entire lengths of their thighs, a choice that befuddled me, considering the voracious mosquitoes which already swarmed us.

To my right stood one such participant who offered up the entirety of her legs to the ravenous, buzzing hordes. She harbored four gargantuan mosquitoes on the side of her leg, their transparent bellies swelling like red balloons as they feasted on her blood. Without so much as looking down, she lobbed a misguided swat in the general direction of the mosquitoes, in the way that a horse's tail blindly swings about its arse to shoo away flies, but none of the mosquitoes flinched.

I considered giving her a friendly heads-up, but before I could formulate my sentence, the gentleman standing across from me arrested my attention. He stood with tall, confident posture, barefoot and shirtless, wearing nothing but a pair of shorts, and a short pair at that. More so than his disregard for mosquitoes, his lack of footwear dumbfounded me. Even with the retreat's well-manicured dirt paths, the idea of going barefoot anywhere in the Amazon jungle boggled my Western mind. Several of the shamans also went barefoot, but they at least wore a protective layer of thick callused flesh that functioned as organic sandals, unlike the delicate, virgin feet of my shirtless cohort.

I diverted my attention by preemptively swatting at the few exposed areas of flesh around my neck and face. Without a word, my shirtless and shoeless cohort wandered off, straight legged and with proper posture, only to return a few minutes later hobbling with a lopsided gait. A small but steady flow of fresh blood trickled out from underneath his big toenail as he mumbled a nonchalant comment about perhaps putting a Band-Aid on it. I offered my silent condolences, and though I didn't understand his thinking, I did envy his ability to shrug off injuries.

After all participants arrived, the staff assigned individual huts to us, with instructions to drop off our luggage and regroup for floral baths. The fresh blister on my foot now forced me to hobble as if wearing a peg leg, toward my hut a few minutes away. Midway there a tall tree caught my attention with its countless long and sharp spines protruding outward in every direction from its trunk, eager to pierce and maim any fleshy creature that dared to come near. The tree's intimidating spines seemed to snarl at me as I stared with eyes aghast, and I cautioned myself to beware of porcupine trees when stumbling through the dark, back to my hut in a loopy Ayahuasca daze.

I swiveled my peg leg up the front steps of my hut, opened the screen door, and then hobbled over to the bed where I sat to inspect the searing blister on my foot. With great caution I slid off my rubber boot, untucked my pajama pant leg from my soggy, sweaty tube sock, then rolled the tube sock downward off

14

my foot to avoid friction on the blister. The jungle symphony faded from my ears as I braced myself to behold the horror of my injury.

A thick flap of wrinkled skin dangled from the ball of my foot, barely clinging to a bright pink slab of raw flesh that glowed with searing pain. The unsightly blister complemented an unrelated wound upon my other foot, which resulted from a bicycle mishap two days prior. So now with two open wounds upon my feet, I had serious reservations about the upcoming floral bath — being doused with water deemed unsafe to drink. Though I didn't know much about infectious diseases, contracting typhoid through the open wounds on my feet seemed like a real possibility, so I hobbled back to the meeting grounds and consulted with a staff member who glanced me over and offered a sincere but unhelpful assertion.

"Nah, you should be fine."

The brief consultation failed to quell my fears, but as I stood in the jungle's gagging humidity and sweltering heat, covered in a sticky blanket of sweat and grime, disgust with myself momentarily eclipsed my fear of infectious diseases. To my own surprise, I followed in the footsteps of my barefoot bleeding-toe friend, and I threw caution to the wind: with open wounds on both feet, I relished in a brisk floral bath of potentially contaminated water. The smiling shamans poured buckets of flower-infused water over my head, and I convinced myself that the sweet-smelling floral agents would somehow protect me from infectious diseases.

Thoughts of typhoid resurfaced as I arrived back at my hut, but I tried to clear my mind by conceding that if I did just infect myself, then the damage was already done, and worrying about it wouldn't help. I dried myself off, put back on the same suit of flannel armor, and then proceeded to the ceremonial hut for orientation.

A thick fog of collective anxiousness hung about the air while the head of staff explained the details of the ceremonies. They would begin promptly at eight o'clock each night, in the massive circular hut in which we currently sat. We would forgo dinner on ceremonial nights, to maximize our stomach's absorption of the brew, and to minimize the mess of vomiting. Our five shamans would sit in the center of the hut, and the twenty of us would sit equidistant from each other in a circle around the circumference of the hut, upon a thin mat equipped with a pillow and vomit pail. One by one we would be summoned to the center to receive our dose.

For the first ceremony, everyone would start with a half dose to gauge our tolerance. For the subsequent ceremonies, we would be free to choose our own dosages. Once everyone had gulped down a dose, the staff would extinguish all lanterns, and the ceremonies would be held in complete darkness. Allowing time for the brew to take effect, we would wait forty-five minutes to an hour in complete silence, in complete darkness, until the shamans began their chanting. After a short prelude from their central position in the hut, they would spread out equidistant among us — the outside circle of participants — sitting face-to-face with us while singing a chant that would, according to Shipibo shamanism, assist us in our journey by summoning benevolent spirits, warding off evil spirits, and so forth.

After the shamans finished their songs, they would lay hands upon us, blowing two forceful gusts of breath, one atop the head, and one between our outstretched hands pressed together — believed to be the two pathways into the soul, or consciousness, or whatever one chooses to call it — which would function as a healing or protective blessing of sorts. The shamans would then scoot over to the next participant and repeat the process of sing, blow, scoot, such that each of us would receive one chant from each of the five shamans as they rotated around the room counterclockwise.

The ceremonies would conclude at midnight, at which time we would be free to stay the night in the ceremonial hut or return to our individual huts. During and after the ceremonies, staff would be on hand to provide physical or psychological support to anyone who may need it.

The staff offered several suggestions to help us through the experience. They advised that some of our visions would potentially be unpleasant or difficult, but that trying to resist them would be counterproductive; the best option was simply to accept it, and to remember that everything passes.

They advised we bring a pillow and blanket for extra comfort because our body temperatures, while staying within a safe range, would be unpredictable.

They advised that diarrhea is a common side effect, and they advised to never trust a fart.

They asked that we be considerate of others by avoiding unnecessary noise, by shielding our flashlights and treading softly if we need to walk to the bathroom, and so forth. But they also advised that if we felt a compelling need to cry or laugh during the ceremony, to go ahead and let it out, while being considerate of others.

Lastly, the staff requested that we try not to vomit on the shamans while they are singing to us.

Our orientation adjourned, and the fog of anxiousness persisted as we disbanded. It persisted as we regrouped for dinner that night — what would be our last dinner for two days — and it persisted as we bid each other a nervous goodnight.

I returned to my hut and lay in bed, relishing in the profound darkness of the nighttime jungle — a welcome change compared to my usual bedroom intrusions from streetlamps and headlights. But despite the idyllic curtain of darkness, despite my sleep deprivation, and despite the exhausting hike, a surging current of excitement and anticipation zapped any trace of sleepiness.

The soft but rapid feet of scurrying lizards zig-zagged across the length of my hut's thatched roof. A fierce wind howled from what sounded like the other end of the earth. The humid aroma of approaching rain, subtle but unmistakable, wafted into my hut and cuddled into bed with me as distant flashes of lightning illuminated the jungle. Ferocious raindrops crashed into the distant jungle canopy and emulated the soft rapping sound of a million fingertips tapping hardcover books. The intensifying deluge marched closer and closer, one thunderous pace at a time, and then stopped directly above to unleash a torrential downpour of majestic aural beauty.

The crushing power of the benevolent tempest squelched my anxiety and quieted my thoughts. Like a loving parent putting her child to bed, Mother Nature caressed my face with backhanded fingertips of cool, stormy breeze, embraced me with the warm sound of terrific rain, and soothed my restless mind, lulling me into peaceful slumber. Though I didn't know it at the time, this would be the final night of my former self.

First Night with Ayahuasca

The nocturnal jungle creatures sang the final movement of their symphony as thin beams of warm sunlight broke through the crevices in the forest canopy. Waking consciousness slowly trickled into my head as I lay motionless, listening to the daytime creatures sing the soft interlude of their symphony. The ambient and soothing sound of their chirps and hoots and croaks and clicks contrasted sharply with civilization's rude awakenings: the honking of morning traffic, the stench and clamor of industrial waste collection, and the nagging screech of alarm clocks.

The fog of dreamland cleared from my mind, leaving only the now-familiar residue of persistent anxiousness. I arose from bed and put on my least favorite long-sleeved shirt, knowing that today I would puke for certain, along with everyone else, because today's agenda started with "stomach cleansing" — a euphemism for self-induced vomiting. To aid us in the endeavor, we first gathered to practice yoga exercises that targeted the upper abdominals and other muscles that would be straining as we retched.

We stood near each other looking ahead at our instructor who demonstrated deft manipulation of her abdominals, rolling her flat stomach in smooth, undulating waves, inflating and deflating it like the throat of a bullfrog. Her impressive feats of physical prowess didn't strike me as something that could be learned in our brief training session, but did seem advantageous for self-induced vomiting.

Without missing a beat in her rhythmic undulations, she smiled at our befuddled faces and encouraged us to join her.

"Okay, now you all try!"

We all tried, and most of us failed. Our clumsy abdomens mostly just shook and jiggled, but two folks in particular stood out. Oddity number one was a middle-aged gentleman who extended his hands outward at waist height, as if gripping a pair of hips, while pumping his crotch back and forth with unintentionally lewd gyrations. I presumed his awkward thrusting must be a subconscious manifestation of his pent-up testosterone, similar to my unintentional and shameful arousal by a faceless mannequin the previous day.

Oddity number two was an older gentleman who, seemingly uninterested in abdominal exercises, took the opportunity to relieve himself of gas. It seeped out at its own pace, neither forced nor restrained, through what sounded like a weathered and weary sphincter. The voluminous plume reeked like eighty-year-old rotten eggs, as did the second plume a few moments later, which he followed up with an audible and unapologetic sigh of relief. His pungent fumes broke the concentration of surrounding participants, most of whom already struggled with the exercises.

We wrote off our losses and commenced the training, then migrated with hesitant feet to the altar of retching: a makeshift wooden bench lined with three plastic bowls and three large water buckets. The staff explained that we would line up three at a time — one person in front of each water bucket — drink a concoction of lemongrass, wait thirty seconds, and then chug water as fast as possible to induce projectile vomiting. Immediately after the vomiting subsided, we would again start chugging water to induce a second projectile vomiting, and then once more for a total of three times.

All three initial participants gulped down the clear lemongrass brew without faltering, and as it swam in their stomachs, no one gave indications of nausea or physical distress — only nervous dread. Each participant cast an uneasy gaze over the altar and off into the jungle as they held their water bowls and awaited the signal to start chugging. No one said a word or made a sound, save for a few prolonged exhales and murmurs of pessimistic speculation from the sidelines. Our only solace came from knowing that we were all on empty stomachs and wouldn't be vomiting up anything solid.

The lead staff member broke the heavy silence with the words no one wanted to hear.

"Okay, start chugging."

Two of the three participants sprung to a valiant start, pouring several bowls of water down their throats nonstop. But as they approached maximum capacity, they slowed their paces to Sunday brunch tea sipping interspersed with premature dry heaving, while the third participant, hesitant from the start, poured water mostly down the sides of his face and neck. All three stared off into the distance, unable to suppress the groans that bubbled out between slow gulps.

Despite his inaccurate pouring, participant number three made the best progress, and mid-gulp he cast his bowl to the side while spewing forth a violent stream of reddish-pink liquid. Everyone's attention turned toward him, and hushed whispers emanated from the crowd of onlookers.

"Did he just...vomit...blood?"

Tea-sipping participant number one lowered her bowl from her mouth and held a hand on her belly as her unfocused eyes bulged in their sockets. She opened her mouth and heaved but spewed forth only a labored groan. She reached the brink of vomiting but then hesitated, and as she lowered her bowl, staff members shouted words of encouragement.

"Keep drinking!"

"You're almost there!"

After bellowing out an exaggerated sigh, she slammed two more large gulps and then secured the silver medal as a mess of liquid erupted from her face. The colorless vomit

21

spraying from her mouth and nose helped to instill confidence in us that participant number three's bloody vomit was not caused by the lemongrass concoction but by personal stomach issues. He himself instilled further confidence in us as he continued to chug and retch two more times, each expulsion less red and less alarming than the previous. He finished all three iterations of vomiting and then strolled off stage with a nonchalant comment directed at no one in particular.

"Huh, my puke was kind of bloody colored. Weird..."

Despite aggressive encouragement from the sidelines, participant number two continued to straggle behind until a staff member leaned in and muttered to him some friendly advice.

"If you don't throw up now, you're going to have bad diarrhea later."

That motivated him to slam four large gulps, after which he immediately heaved it all out.

As I watched the nine participants in front of me chug and spew and chug and spew, most of them struggling and miserable, I took note of one fellow who aced the entire process like a seasoned professional. On his triumphant victory stroll back to the herd, I pulled him aside to ask if he had any advice, and it turned out that he did indeed.

"Pretty simple, really. When you hit the point where you feel like you can't drink any more, that's when you drink more."

I kept that in mind as two more participants toiled through the process and my turn came. Despite the projectile nature of everyone's vomiting, the tail end of it fell to the ground in front of them, followed by a steady dribble onto their shoes, shirts, and chins. By the time I stepped up to the altar, the accumulation of saliva and regurgitated lemongrass water had soaked the ground into a soggy mess.

The staff handed me a bowl of lemongrass water, and I sampled a small sip, surprised that it lacked any strong flavor. The entire bowlful glided down my throat with ease, and as I reached for the large water bowl sitting upon the altar, I wondered about the sanitary risk of twenty strangers sharing the same three unwashed bowls potentially contaminated with each other's vomit. In my hands I held the same bowl used by participant number three, whose bloody vomit cast further doubt upon the hygienic integrity of the operation.

I deliberated whether to raise the issue, but in a scatterbrained fit of pre-vomit jitters, I managed to console myself by assuming that I probably already got typhoid from the floral bath, and that would cancel out whatever diseases had splattered onto the bowl. Before I could scrutinize that questionable logic, the staff announced commencement of the round.

"All right, drink!"

An unexpected rush of motivation took over me as I slammed the first two bowls of water, barely taking time to breathe. My stomach stretched to uncomfortable proportions, heavy with the weight of water, while the staff cheered us on.

"Good, good. Keep going."

My natural instincts demanded that I stop, now at the point where I felt like I couldn't drink anymore, but I pressed on as the professional vomiting champion's advice still echoed in my mind.

Mid-chug, the water going down my throat suddenly switched directions, and before I could move the bowl out of the way, I threw up back into it, strengthening my suspicions that I was not the first to do so. After forcing out the last drops from my stomach, I poured another deluge of water down my throat until my stomach once again ejected all its contents onto the

23

muddy ground in front of me. A female shaman standing behind me offered moral support, patting me on the back as I caught my breath. Her pantomimes instructed me to slam three more bowls and then stick two fingers down my throat, which forced out my final spew. The shaman massaged a thick and stubby knuckle into my lower abdominals, coaxing out the last few dribbles before she accepted my futile dry heaving as evidence that I was empty.

It had been two years since my previous vomiting, which also happened to be projectile, but on that occasion I shot out of my face a wine-soaked, partially digested gluttonous mess of spicy Indian curry with naan. On this occasion, my self-induced projectile vomiting of clear water proved much more manageable, unpleasant only in the initial bloating, and what I had dreaded to be a long and miserable process turned out to be short and tolerable.

The pride of surmounting that psychological hurdle faded as I honed my attention on the next, much steeper hurdle — my impending immersion into the unknown depths of my subconscious. My racing thoughts throughout the day all blurred together, leaving me with no memories other than vague excerpts of breakfast, lunch, lounging around in hammocks, and skipping my floral bath.

My nervous excitement intensified with each passing hour as the ceremony drew nearer, as the sun ducked further out of sight, and as the jungle symphony transitioned back to the nighttime creatures. The fading aura of dusk barely illuminated the jungle path as I made my way toward the ceremonial hut, pillow and blanket in hand, and in passing I casted a leery stare at the deadly spines of the porcupine tree.

At the ceremonial hut's entrance, I discarded my shoes — the only pair in sight — next to a disorderly mountain of sandals, then walked up the short flight of wooden stairs leading inside. Insect-proof screening encompassed the hut, and the nighttime's encroaching darkness consumed all but the faint glow of lanterns inside. No one spoke a word as the creaking of footsteps and the soft rustling of cloth emanated outward from the hut, along with a musk of collective nervousness.

The door whimpered a soft creak as I nudged it open and peered inside. A symmetric arrangement of dim lanterns illuminated the room only enough to see body-length mats lining the outer edge of the circular hut. Each mat rested equidistant from its neighbor, meticulously spaced in a circle resembling the sarcophagus layout of a grand mausoleum. At the edge of each sarcophagus rested a vomit pail for a headstone, its epitaph waiting to be written in the fresh vomit of the departed. The headstones pointed toward the mausoleum's center, comprised of the five sarcophagi and unmarked headstones of our shamans, who would not only guide us but also join us on our departure from this world.

I tiptoed along the perimeter toward my sarcophagus, passing the anonymous silhouettes of my cohorts. In a flash of nervous paranoia, it struck me that this setting — strong spiritual overtones guiding a fringe group's ritualistic gathering and drinking of a concoction — bore an uncomfortable resemblance to that of a mass suicide.

The thin mat of my sarcophagus provided minimal cushioning and limited options as I tried to ascertain the most comfortable position for dying. I settled into a half lotus and sat through grueling minutes of silence as we awaited the arrival of our shamans. My nervous attempts at last-minute mental preparation flip-flopped between self-assurance and self-sabotage, and my mind raced as the shamans trickled in one by one.

The fifth and final shaman stepped into the mausoleum, greeting us with a low and barely audible "buenas noches" as she took her seat in the center. The head of staff signaled with a subtle hand gesture for participant number one to approach the shamans, and we all watched him lurch toward the altar wearing a nervous smile that accented rather than veiled his anxiety. He sat face-to-face with the lead shaman, then adjusted and readjusted his posture several times in the span of a few seconds. The shaman poured a dose and handed the tiny glass to him, and all eyes in the room fixated on his labored gulp and his clenched eyelids as the thick, dark-brown liquid swam out of the glass and down his throat.

He grimaced and handed the glass back to the shaman while offering a forced smile and a nod of gratitude. His bare feet pressed against the wooden floorboards as he tiptoed back to his sarcophagus, with a quick shudder and cringe. Each successive participant followed suit, lurching to the altar, choking down a tiny glassful of dark-brown elixir, and then cringing during their nervous shuffle back.

Even though I knew Ayahuasca was safe when administered properly, the nearest hospital was three hours away — by foot, by boat, and then by bus — which fueled a sudden outbreak of loud and irrational worries in my mind. But as my turn approached, the absence of adverse reactions in the first dozen participants helped calm my fears. And given that I had only seven nights with Ayahuasca, part of me argued that I should dive in headfirst and start with a full dose, rather than waste one night on a small dose.

I took my seat at the altar and stared at the Ayahuasca contained inside an ancient relic of a plastic bottle permanently stained dark brown from years of use. From up close the brew resembled motor oil, and the grotesque sight of it vanquished my ambitions of starting with a full dose.

The shaman poured my dose, and I watched the glugging with the same dread and anxiety of watching a doctor prepare a syringe. The shaman handed the dose to me and nodded "go ahead" as I took the glass into my hand. Rather than shooting it straight away as all my predecessors had, I inhaled a hearty whiff of the brew first. While holding the cup to my nostrils and absorbing the bitter odor, I looked up at the shaman, whose stern gaze of disbelief clued me in to the rudeness of my altar manners.

During my early twenties, multiple failed attempts at drinking shots of alcohol had proven that I cannot quickly drink distasteful liquids, so I divided the Ayahuasca dose into two small gulps. A foul wave of bitterness assaulted my palette, biting with an acrid sting that coated my mouth and followed the brew all the way down my throat and into my belly. The shaman's unwavering gaze shifted from disbelief to consolation, as if to say, "I know it tastes like battery acid, but it'll be worth it." I squinted and tried to force a smile, realized that I couldn't muster one, and instead nodded in gratitude.

The relentless bitterness clung to my taste buds as I shuffled back to my sarcophagus. My every breath reeked of Ayahuasca's nauseating stench, repeatedly reminding me of the nastiness churning in my belly. I returned to half lotus position on my mat, closed my eyes to avoid the sight of others struggling through their doses, and then pulled my vomit pail nearer, convinced that I might need it.

After ten minutes the nausea receded, plateauing at a manageable level. The warm glow of the hut's lanterns began to fade, and I opened my eyes to see the staff extinguishing the lanterns one by one until the entire room vanished into pitch black. I couldn't see my own hands in front of me. No one in the room made a sound — no coughing or mumbling or clearing of throats or cracking of knuckles — and the deafening silence supplanted the jungle symphony still playing in the background.

My attention turned inward as I closed my eyes and reminded myself of my two main focal points for the ceremonies: my recent career change from IT to writing, and a painful breakup from the past that still weighed heavy on me. The staff's advice also echoed in my head, reminding me to accept whatever may come, no matter how unpleasant.

My stomach blurted out a confused moan, leery of the new and unfamiliar liquid, flabbergasted as to how something so foul had managed to pass through the filtering system of my taste buds. I sealed my lips to stifle a series of short belches that bubbled up, each one reminding me of Ayahuasca's vile taste.

An unfamiliar anxiety crept through my body, distinct from the psychologically induced variety that plagued me thus far. This new strain of anxiety felt chemically induced, and though subtle at first, it gradually intensified until forcing me to adjust my seated position.

Blurry but colorful geometric patterns emerged behind my closed eyes, like a rudimentary kaleidoscope coming into focus. Sunbursts of pastel radii intersected a waterfall of cascading triangles and diamonds, all interwoven on a soothing backdrop of warm and cool colors that swam like schools of jellyfish, entrancing in their beautiful and unpredictable motions. The brilliant visuals instilled tranquility within me, vanquishing my anxiety as they captivated my attention like a mobile hanging above a baby's crib, and I, like an infant, marveled at the slow-motion fireworks.

My jaw began to dance on its own, subtle at first, shifting left and right in four-four time to the slow beat of imaginary music. The unconscious jaw movements soon moseyed into my awareness, and I began rocking back and forth, likewise feeling the same beat of imaginary music and feeling compelled to move with it. But sitting upright felt tiresome and unnatural, and fatigue soon overwhelmed me. I opened my eyes to find a thin layer of the kaleidoscope patterns overlaid on top of the hut's darkness, and the room began to spin.

From sitting position, I leaned back onto my hands, and they walked themselves farther backward, lowering my torso in a slow descent. The vile liquid in my stomach shifted as I lay horizontally, and the inner lining of my stomach, now highly sensitive, relayed to me in exquisite detail the precise motion, depth, and location of the Ayahuasca as its tiny waves swayed back and forth inside me. A chill ran through me, extinguishing the warmth of the summer jungle, and when I pulled my blanket over my legs, they felt detached and unfamiliar, as if they had fallen asleep, but without tingling or numbness.

A comforting wave of relief rushed through me as I lay on my back, no longer concerned with the arduous chore of balancing myself upright, and no longer burdened with the increasingly foreign notion of having a physical body. All my muscles relaxed, and my consciousness drifted away from my physical body, discarding the unnecessary vessel like a snake shedding skin.

The kaleidoscope visions transitioned into plantlike visions of lush jungle vegetation. The light browns of tree trunks and branches melded with the brilliant greenery of their leaves and a web of vines, complementing a picturesque blue sky that peeked through from behind. The plant life comprised three-dimensional, living wallpaper that lined the insides of a silo in which I found myself. The organic walls swayed in a calm breeze, extending up vertically farther than I could see, fading into a warm glow of gorgeous white light from above.

Down from the infinite heights of the silo descended a thick green vine with smooth, vibrant, glistening textures that radiated health and vitality. From the tip of the vine sprouted a head resembling a Venus flytrap, which guided the vine as it slithered down with the slow and powerful grace of a python, stopping just above my face as I gazed up in awe. The outer rim of its soft, toothless mouth clapped together in anticipation, and a curious, mutual desire for contact swarmed between us.

The python vine stretched its jaw open wider, than my face, eclipsing the brilliant light from above, and I closed my eyes and bowed my head, signaling to the python vine to descend upon me. Its soft and toothless gums gently clamped down and gnawed on my head like a puppy playing with a chew toy. Dozens of finger-length flagella massaged my scalp and lulled me into a trance, and I basked in a state of blissful awe, unable to contain my giggling. The scalp massage evolved into a symbiotic relationship, with the python vine feeding off electrified, life-giving nutrients emanating from my noggin, selectively extracting only my surplus sustenance so as not to deplete me.

I pressed my tongue against the back of my teeth and gums, which felt foreign like when numbed by a dentist's anesthesia, except with my sense of touch heightened rather than dulled. Neither my gums nor my teeth felt like they belonged to me, yet the tactile sensations registered in my consciousness. Familiarity with my lips likewise faded away, and new visions precipitated behind my closed eyes as my tongue and jaw danced on their own.

From a third-person perspective, I saw myself standing on the outskirts of an unfamiliar city, my body facing toward a distant horizon of skyscrapers. An inexplicable confusion disoriented me until I realized that the entire vision appeared upside down like a television turned on its head. Flocks of inverted bird silhouettes beat their wings upward, soaring across a purple-blue sky below me, while a sidewalk stretched overhead, comprising the ceiling from which my body hung upside down like a bat. My observing consciousness tried to correct the vision by flipping it right side up, but the background remained fixed and only my body spun right side up, floating like a superimposed cutout upon the upside-down background. Confusion intensified as I stared at my motionless body with its feet standing upon the dark sky, while the pointed tops of skyscrapers dangled from above like stalactites.

A lighthearted exhale seeped out as I gave up on correcting the vision. In letting go of my desire for control, a peaceful stillness took over, allowing me to detect a signal — a nonverbal but energized invitation calling to me from the city. It beckoned me to come explore, and a childlike curiosity compelled me toward the stalactite skyscrapers in the distance. But as I watched myself take steps forward, the city moved farther away, retreating behind the horizon. The faster my body walked toward the city, the faster the city retreated.

From across the hut, a sudden death cry of involuntary gurgling and dry heaving shattered the silence of the room and startled me back into the physical world. The ordeal sounded less like vomiting and more like an exorcism: the heaving sounds launched upward from an abyss far deeper than his stomach, as if a dense clump of parasitic evil clung to the walls of his intestines; its heinous screeching reverberated up the length of his digestive tract as his body strained to expel the affliction. Each bloodcurdling heave started with a low tremble, resonating with deep bass that wavered and cracked as the pitch of his cries traversed two entire octaves. His desperate body sounded unconcerned with potentially vomiting up his entire digestive tract as collateral damage. Each heave grew longer and scarier than the last, and his gurgling death cries mutated into prolonged fits of frantic straining, as if he were giving oral birth to a gargantuan clump of viscous agony. After several minutes of straining, his body collapsed and spilled forth a protracted epilogue of groaning, whimpering, and exasperated sighs of relief, until finally his murmurs faded into a requiem of silence.

As I lay on my back, a sudden compulsion implored me to rise into sitting position. I propped myself up with weary arms,

31

and my head began to sway on its own to imaginary music, as if entranced by a snake charmer. My torso likewise followed suit, and my knees began to flap like the wings of a fledgling bird. My face turned upward as if pulled from behind, and I gasped through my nostrils.

An exotic intoxication of intimidating strength nudged my hands off the reins of my consciousness and secured a firm grip of its own. Ayahuasca seized me like a living, sentient, intelligent organism imposing its mind control over me and forcibly taking possession of my body. Though I maintained a lucid connection to my consciousness, the dominating possession of Ayahuasca usurped my psychological sovereignty, ousting me as the former ruler of my consciousness, relegating me to a meek and humble peasant observing from the sidelines of my lowly rank.

The exhilarating intoxication gripped me with its benevolent but unfathomable power as I quivered and squirmed in delight. Profound reverence paralyzed me with stunning awe and humility, and my mind raced to find a memory of any past astonishment comparable in magnitude. Brief flashbacks of awe-inspiring experiences flickered in my mind — beholding the beauty and stillness of the earth's vast mountain ranges, beholding the sky set ablaze as the sun sinks into a horizon of rolling ocean waves likewise set ablaze, beholding thousands of twinkling stars on a clear night sky while trying to grasp the infinite vastness of the cosmos — but they all paled in comparison to the otherworldly awe raging through me.

The intensity of such a small dose flabbergasted me, and I failed to formulate even a basic mental reaction, slurring my intended thought of "¡Ay, caramba!" into "¡Ay, yahuasca!"

Before my closed eyes, two naked bodies appeared, clasped together in a passionate embrace, throbbing with carnal desire. They buried their faces in the other's neck as they groped and kneaded gluttonous handfuls of each other, but I recognized them as myself and my ex-girlfriend, floating in darkness, without so much as a bed to lie on. Their two naked bodies — the only two objects in the universe, endlessly gravitating into each other — floated through dark, empty space, and their limbs intertwined to form one gyrating organism that pulsated with a golden glow of passion.

As I watched from a third-person perspective, my body relayed all its tactile sensations to me in real time, in high fidelity. I watched myself gently kissing her neck, and I felt her pulse on my lips, the rapid beating of her racing heart. I watched her straddling me just above the waist, and I felt the smooth warmth of her soft inner thighs pressed against me. I watched her lowering her hips to align our parts, and I felt the thin trail of moisture that she smeared down my abdomen. I watched myself slide inside her.

My own sharp inhale startled me out of the vision as I trembled, overwhelmed by the tangible sensation of sexual penetration.

Intimate memories of her played before my eyes in a rapid-fire montage. Disjointed scenes flashed by like a spliced movie reel in fast forward — graphic depictions of us ravaging each other's bodies, close-ups of her clenched eyelids and mouth agape as she approached climax, her trembling thighs wrapped around my waist, the bulging veins in my embracing arms as I clamped our sweaty bodies together.

The vision captivated me on a primal level, but at the same time felt empty and salacious, and my higher consciousness implored me to better utilize the opportunity for something more meaningful than immersive pornography. The retreat's prohibition of all sexual activity — even between husbands and wives — resurfaced in my mind, and an awkward blend of fear and shame further implored me to avoid pitching a tent.

My eyelids opened but I saw only darkness as I placed my thumbs on my temples and rubbed my forehead with the remaining eight digits, helping to reset my mental state. One of my distant neighbors also helped to reset my mental state by seemingly vomiting up his entire stomach. Like falling dominos, his furious heaving triggered vomiting in another neighbor, creating a fortuitous ensemble of wretched gurgling noises that wiped away all my erotic thoughts in one grand swoop.

Throughout my life, the sight or sound or smell of vomiting had always nauseated me, so I had gone into the ceremony with serious concerns about such disturbances detracting from my experience. But as I sat front row in the circus of vomiting, I decided that rather than resisting the sounds, I would focus on them, and in the instant when I switched from resistance to acceptance, I nearly exploded with laughter. My chest convulsed and I clasped both hands over my mouth to stifle the laughter which, if it blurted out, would have sounded callous and diabolical. The hilarity stemmed not from anyone's misery, but from the objective sound of such ridiculous noises gushing from trembling orifices.

The head shaman, indifferent to the retching of my neighbors, scooted in front of me and signaled the start of his chant by shooting a series of powerful breaths through the blowgun barrel of his closed hands.

Rather than darting at me in a straight line from the shaman's lips to my ears, the sounds of his breath swirled through the room like howling specters. My heightened sense of hearing served as a fine-tuned sonar system, and despite interference from the circus of vomiting, I tracked the nimble dance of the specters through the air before they dove at me in pirouettes from unpredictable angles.

The vomiting baritones continued wailing their wretched duet, and I continued suppressing my inappropriate laughter. The head shaman concluded his prelude of breaths, transitioning to a hum of powerful bass that vibrated in my chest, followed by a serenade of lyrics sung in his native Shipibo language. Though he sat three body lengths away and sang with a soft, mumbling voice, his song resonated with such startling clarity and volume that I swore he sat close enough to kiss my ears.

The second male shaman faded in with his own unique chant which complemented the head shaman's, and their duet of soothing vibrations escorted me back to the world of Ayahuasca visions.

On a black backdrop of empty space, a porcupine tree materialized before me, exuding a dark cloud of malicious intent, menacing like a predator lying in wait, and beaming with vivid realism which surpassed that of the actual porcupine tree along the jungle path. The long needle-like spines glistened as if salivating to pierce my flesh, and a gruesome premonition flashed before me: that I would die upon these spines. My intuition knew it to be true, and the dread of my imminent mangling paralyzed me. In a panic I tried to conjure up a baseball bat with which I could destroy the spines, but I then took a deep breath and reminded myself of the staff's advice. I acknowledged the futility in trying to fight or run, I fixed my gaze directly at the spines, I accepted that they were meant for my flesh, and I conceded my fate of death by porcupine tree.

One at a time, the three female shamans converged into the chorus of chants, and their voices lashed at my ears with sharp, sour dissonance. They boomed with the same astounding power as the male shamans, but rather than complementing each other, they clashed like a trio of ramshackle violins, out of tune and off-key.

The porcupine tree salivated in silence, and I felt my physical body detaching from my consciousness. I watched the back of my head emerge into my field of vision as my body stepped forward and left my observing consciousness behind. I watched my body march with confident steps toward the porcupine tree, stopping just shy of the thousands of spines protruding from its trunk. I watched myself size up the porcupine tree and then take a final enthusiastic step forward with open arms, face first into the spines, embracing the lethal trunk like a dear friend.

Like darts to a bull's-eye, two spines pierced through the clear concave corneas of my eyeballs, tearing into the blacks of my irises. Blood flowed like tears from my eyes as the spines pushed deeper. My detached consciousness zoomed in as the outer layers of my physical body faded into transparency and displayed in hyper-vivid detail the spines stabbing out of the backsides of my eyeballs, piercing into the soft, spongy tissue of my brain. Other spines pierced my nose, sliding through my nasal cavity, likewise stabbing into my brain. A melee of countless more spines splintered and snapped to pieces as they crushed up against my teeth and against the bones of my cheeks and forehead.

My gruesome death unfolded before me, but I felt no pain and no emotion other than reluctant acceptance as I mumbled to myself.

"So this is how I die..."

Dozens of spines lacerated my throat, and each of my body's labored attempts at inhalation drew in as much blood as air. The longest spines tore through my chest, finding the gaps in my rib cage, stabbing through my slowly beating heart and through my lungs. A battalion of long and short spines maimed the soft flesh of my abdomen, stabbing through my innards and protruding out my lower back. A brownish-red mixture of blood and feces seeped out from the holes in my flesh, dripping from the tips of the tree's unbroken needles. Merciless spines skewered my genitals, several through each testicle and several lengthwise through the head and shaft of my flaccid member, pinning it against my inner thigh.

My detached consciousness zoomed out for a wider view of my decimated, transparent corpse impaled on the porcupine tree. I watched my lifeless body fall limp as blood streaked down my clear torso with such vivid realism that, without questioning reality, I accepted that I had indeed died. My detached visual perspective and my intimate familiarity with my own body combined into a strange sense that I had not only witnessed but also experienced my own death, and with a calm voice I delivered my own succinct eulogy.

"Now I'm dead."

The words triggered a flash of lucidity, and for the first time in my life, I fully accepted my mortality. This new acceptance exposed my stealthy self-sabotage — my lifelong denial and avoidance of death — and the accumulated burden of repressed grief that I had been carrying for my entire adult life. The epiphany instantly liberated me from my fear of death, and it diffused a suffocating mental pressure that had always weighed down on me but which I had grown accustomed to and written off as normal.

My limp body hung impaled on the porcupine tree like a victim of self-crucifixion, but from my detached perspective I peered through the blood-soaked forest of spines that mutilated my face, and I saw my lacerated lips and cheeks widen into a peaceful smile of content.

A sudden and powerful exhale jarred me back into the physical world as the second male shaman finished his one-on-one with my neighbor next door. Dreadful fatigue fought me in my attempt to sit up straight, but I managed to rise victorious as the shaman scooted over to me. He remained invisible in the pitch black of night, and I tracked his movements by the sound of his plastic vomit pail sliding across the planks of the uneven wooden floor, followed by the soft thud of his hind parts plopping down in front of me.

I listened for the faint sound of his lips parting to signal the start of his chant, but without warning his mighty singing voice slammed against my torso like a gale force wind, and the powerful beauty of his voice instantly entranced me. My body involuntarily swayed from side to side, and my jaw improvised a two-step jig to the beat of his melody, amplifying the passion with which I listened. Though he and I shared no spoken language, hadn't made any physical contact, and couldn't even see each other's face, he sang to me with the sincerity and intimacy of a father singing to his only son.

He concluded with a euphoric outro that slowly faded into silence, but the power of his song continued to resonate inside me. The floorboards creaked beneath the weight of his feet as he rose to stand and bestow a blessing upon me. He rested his hands upon my unwashed head to orient himself, then slurped up a small mouthful of scented water. His curled hands formed a makeshift blowgun with which he blew a cool wet gust of breath onto the top of my head. His wet hands then slid down my neck and shoulders in search of my outstretched arms. The soft leathery flesh of his wet fingertips grazed against my hands as he found his grip, pressing my palms together and sandwiching them between his own. With the precision of a master craftsman, he positioned my fingertips on the cusp of his bottom lip and wedged my palms apart just enough to allow the passage of air. His nostrils drew in a deep inhale, and then his lips blew an emphatic gust of wet, scented breath that traversed the confines of my wedged palms and my outstretched arms.

The gust of breath infiltrated my chest with unwavering momentum, spreading throughout my torso and filling me with satisfying warmth like hot chocolate on a frigid winter night.

My arms remained extended in gratitude, and we both sat in silence for a moment before he patted the tops of my palms to signal "all done". He then scooted off while whispering a few syllables in his native Shipibo language, unintelligible to me, but delightful nonetheless.

As soon as I reclined onto my back, the intoxication thrust me into the world of visions.

From a third-person perspective I saw myself standing face-to-face with my ex-girlfriend, both of us fully clothed, with the clarity and immersive realism of the physical world. We stood an arm's length away as we looked into each other's eyes with the same mellow gaze with which we had greeted each other upon waking each morning, still entangled and disheveled from the night before.

Neither of us moved, or even blinked. Emotionless and without a word, still staring into her eyes, I suddenly clenched my right hand into a rock-solid fist, raised it to shoulder height and plunged it into her chest, smashing through her brittle rib cage. The force of the blow launched thick chunks of her bloody flesh into the air as my knuckles tore through her delicate body. Involuntary spasms contorted her face into a twitching grimace of shock and agony as I ground my fist deeper inside her chest, spread open my fingers and grabbed a hold of her heart. Its tough, muscular walls struggled against the tight grip of my stranglehold. She convulsed in excruciating pain as I yanked out her beating heart, the elastic arteries snapping like rubber bands, one by one in quick succession. I held up her heart at eye level, and showers of blood squirted out to the rhythm of her frantic heartbeat, splattering my face and hers. A steady stream of blood ran down my forearm and dripped off my elbow into a pool on the ground as we both stood in silence, hers from speechlessness, mine from cold indifference.

My stern eye contact held steady as I threw her convulsing heart at our feet, and it smashed into the ground with the squishy thud of a ripe tomato. The blood splatter painted our shoes red, matching her blood-soaked shirt, her mangled chest, and my bloodstained arm. Pools of blood coagulated into thick clumps of dark crimson mud at our feet. My indifference silently screamed at her as she looked back at me with trembling eyes, soggy with tears and disbelief. I raised my right knee to waist height, and without even looking down to aim, I stomped her heart with all my strength, over and over, digging my heel into the sinewy mess of bloody tissue, twisting and grinding to wring out every drop.

Tears flowed from her devastated eyes and coalesced with the blood splatters on her face, drawing erratic streaks of pink down her cheeks. Her shattered ribs protruded from the gaping hole in her chest, which still showered me with blood as I broke eye contact for the first time, turned my back, and walked away without a word. She stood frozen in place, blindsided and devastated, unmoving except for her sulking shoulders, which heaved up and down with sharp breaths of silent, uncontrollable sobbing. Hysteria petrified her, and she couldn't even wipe the streaming tears from her face as I disappeared into the darkness, never once looking back at her.

My ego butted in from the sidelines, with a vehement objection.

"OH, COME ON! The breakup wasn't that bad! I did my best to let her down easy!"

I wholeheartedly believed it to be true, that I had done my best to end the relationship painlessly, but the calm and rational voice of my conscience disagreed.

"Maybe it wasn't that bad for you, but that's how it felt for her."

The irrefutable truth hit me in the chest like a sledgehammer, tearing into me with the same ruthless violence with which I had torn into her, and I winced in pain at the realization of my abysmal selfishness. The cloak of egocentrism disintegrated, revealing for the first time the obvious and awful emotional damage that I had inflicted on her, and it broke my heart that I had broken her heart.

Tears welled up beneath my closed eyelids and filled the shallow reservoirs to the brim before spilling out from the corners of my eyes. I lost track of time as a steady flow of tears trickled down my cheeks, but the heart-wrenching devastation within me served as more than just fruitless suffering; it provided emotional manure that, despite its unpleasantness, fertilized a garden of self-improvement, because the vision compelled me to shed my self-centeredness, to burst my inflated ego, to fill the void with empathy, and to never hurt anyone like that again.

Thoughts and reflections streamed through my mind for an unknown span of time until I noticed too late that the next shaman had already sang to me and moved on to my neighbor. Insurmountable fatigue prohibited me from sitting up anyway, so I simply stayed on my back, and a new vision unfolded.

A voluptuous young woman with the proportions of a goddess floated before me on a background of moving, breathing vegetation. In dazzling detail and realism, the smooth, bronze landscape of her naked body radiated a golden aura like the corona of the setting sun, and her long, black hair swayed behind her weightlessly in unseen currents of primal sexual energy. Her gaze doused me in a warm, electric bath of irresistible lust that melted away my higher consciousness, leaving me with only a speechless physical body driven by

41

insatiable carnal instincts. Her amorous brown eyes flared with desire and beckoned me to come closer.

I floated nearer, holding steady eye contact that advertised the reciprocal desire burning within me. A thick mist of pheromones exuded from my body and piqued her arousal, triggering thousands of long porcupine-tree spines that erupted outward from beneath her soft skin and covered the surface of her body like a sea urchin. But unlike the malevolent spines of the porcupine tree, which had salivated to maim my flesh, her spines shimmered with innocent lust. I sensed through wordless intuition her true nature, that of a loving and benevolent creature tragically cursed with lethal anatomy that banished her to a chaste eternity of unfulfilled desire. Heartfelt sympathy stoked the flames of my burning lust as her deadly beauty possessed me. I advanced within arm's reach, unfazed by her coat of spines, as her amiable eyes widened in surprise. She watched me break eye contact and lower my gaze to the curving V-shape of her bountiful inner thighs, where a dense concentration of spines surrounded her opening. Animal lust deranged my thoughts, and I saw the spines not as a deterrent but simply as the cost of doing business.

I reached with slow and deliberate hands to embrace the wild curves of her hips, and I watched the sharp spines sink into my palms. The needle-thin tips widened at the base, ripping larger and larger holes the deeper they sank into my flesh. They punctured my tendons and muscles without any pain, and I watched unconcerned as they tore out of the backs of my hands. Blood poured forth as the warmth of my impaled palms descended upon her hips, melding our body heat together. She purred with uncontainable arousal, triggering dozens more spines that elongated and pierced the insides of my wrists, rupturing arteries and snapping ligaments, pushing out through the back sides as easily as they had pierced the front.

Her sturdy spines harpooned my hands and wrists as I clamped my wide-fingered grip onto the soft mounds of her hips and pulled her nearer. She floated weightlessly toward me, parting her legs with eager anticipation, and in the valley between her upper thighs, the dense forest of spines elongated and proliferated before my eyes. She spread her thighs wide enough to part the forest of spines and narrowly allow my member a clear pathway into her opening, but as I docked my waist between her legs, hundreds of spines stabbed into my sides and hips. She reached down and grazed her benign fingertips along the underside of my erection as it arrived unscathed at the smooth folds of her lips. We stared into each other's eyes, mutually trembling in anticipation of the moment, and with a soft tug she pleaded for penetration.

I broke eye contact and watched her fingertips safely guide me into her opening, which shimmered from glowing moisture that accentuated her body's golden aura. In slow motion I pushed forward and slid myself further inside her, unconcerned with the thousands of spines decimating my body. Her opening swallowed me, and the hyper-realism of the sleek, enveloping warmth jolted my entire body into a rigid convulsion of ecstasy.

An involuntary gasp pulled me out of the vision as my astounded eyes shot open and darted about the blackness of the room in disbelief. I tried to gulp but choked on the attempt, then clamped my eyes back shut.

Her spines pierced my waist and my hips, sinking deeper into me as I sank deeper into her. She moaned an irrepressible exhale that resonated with a lifetime of unfulfilled desire. Her flesh and spines faded to iridescent transparency — predominantly clear but marbled with rainbow colors like a soap bubble — giving a detailed anatomical view of her insides. The transparent layers of her lower abdomen revealed my member filling her narrow canal as it expanded to accommodate my girth. Only halfway through the initial thrust of penetration, the warm sensation of her moist friction drove me mad with pleasure, like an unwavering plateau of sustained orgasm.

I clasped a hand over my gaping mouth, too late to squelch a sharp gasp that escaped as I writhed on my mat.

My prolonged initial thrust left me breathless and trembling as I watched her clear flesh engulf my entire length. My loins pressed flush against hers, and I froze in awe, marveling at the sublime sight of her warm insides enveloping me. But in that same moment, a cold shiver of dread shot through me, my stomach sank, and I choked on a thick, ominous cloud of immediate danger.

In the flash of a nanosecond, dozens of long, downward-facing spines shot out from her moist inner walls, triggered like the stingers of jellyfish tentacles. Countless spines tore through the swollen head of my erection and lengthwise through my engorged shaft. Shock and dismay arrested me as I gazed through her transparent loins, at the internal mesh of crisscrossed spines piercing my erection. She purred and moaned while my blood streamed out from her lips, down my scrotum and down my legs.

I raised my stupefied gaze from the grisly sight and looked into her amorous eyes, which still glowed with insatiable and innocent passion. She silently begged me to stay, latching a desperate grip around my waist with her spiny legs, sinking the long thorns of her calves into my lower back. She ensnared me like helpless prey caught in a python's bite, and I knew the futility of struggling. Even if I could have escaped, her yearning eyes devastated me, and I couldn't bear to disappoint her, to tease her with a morsel of erotic ecstasy, only to then cast her back into the cold loneliness of eternal solitude.

My psychological arousal withered but my physical arousal held strong. A bewildering but dutiful sense of obligation compelled me to satiate her long-unfulfilled lust, so I concided my morbid fate and slowly slid in and out of her with my bleeding erection, still fully engorged, riddled with stab wounds. Each outward withdrawal provided a moment of reprieve as my erection slid off the spines, and each inward thrust further lacerated me as the spines tore back in. She erupted with heavy moaning to the rhythm of my thrusting, and she reveled in rapturous, long-awaited gratification as I silently watched my own decimation through the clear, iridescent flesh of her loins. Her emphatic moaning motivated me to prolong our gory affair if I could, but within seconds her internal spines shredded my erection into long, stringy strands of useless bloody flesh, and the vision faded to black.

My consciousness seeped back into the physical space behind my eyes and reestablish its connection with my physical body, like a slow and natural waking from dreamland. Next door, invisible in the dark, a female shaman belted out the last verses of her song for my neighbor. I hoisted myself up to sitting position in preparation for her serenade, unsure how many shamans had already passed me by. An unfamiliar nausea — distinct from the urge to vomit, but equally unpleasant — spread throughout my stomach and abdomen, and I reached for my vomit pail as a precaution. A flood of gases and juices sloshed through my digestive tract, filling the nooks and crannies newly opened by my vertical posture. A short series of uncomfortable gurgles and belches helped relieve my nausea, and after a few minutes I returned my unused vomit pail off to the side.

A confusing sobriety dominated me as I sat upright in the darkness. My previously haywire sense of hearing now felt precise, pinpointing the locations of the five singing shamans. My train of thought progressed in coherent, linear fashion. My consciousness resynchronized with my physical body, and I realized that in the heat trapped under my unnecessary blanket, a sticky layer of perspiration covered me. The abrupt return to

45

sobriety convinced me that I needed a stronger dose, and restlessness took over as I wondered when the ceremony would end.

The shaman next door squawked out a shrill melody that oscillated out of key in both directions, and she paused occasionally to choke on globs of phlegm. Her weathered vocal cords struggled, presumably worn down from decades of screeching out her sandpaper song. She concluded with a trailing whimper and a cough, barely mustering the final blowing of breath.

She scooted across the floorboards and pawed to find her position in front of my mat, and I braced myself for a piercing lullaby as she filled her lungs with a massive inhale.

Her song socked me in the face with an initial note of shrieking falsetto that trembled as she struggled to hold it. She then aimed for and completely missed several more excruciating notes even further out of her range. My ears quivered at her jarring shrieks, which sounded less like a song and more like the cries of a dying banshee. I unconsciously reeled back in defense, but the sour tones of her raspy voice chased me down. My face pinched up in disgust as I squirmed in my seat, begging for a hasty end to the torture, and my body initiated a self-defense mechanism that I had never experienced before: my sense of hearing degraded into a muffled mess as if I were underwater, partially numbing the pain.

But soon an epiphany struck, and I remembered that I had to accept the predicament, rather than fight it. With a deep breath I leaned in toward her, forcing myself face-first into the bombardment of wretched harpy shrieks. My muffled hearing cleared up, my quivering ears relaxed, my resistance softened into acceptance, and I heard past her floundering melody and raspy voice. I heard beauty in the passion with which she sang: the beauty of a stranger who didn't know me at all, who didn't even share a common language with me, but who sang her heart out in a strenuous effort to help her fellow human being.

My initial feelings of repulsion melted away into utmost gratitude, and for the remainder of her song I unconsciously swayed back and forth, listening with undivided attention. She concluded her song for me in the same way that she had for my neighbor — with a whimpering outro that trailed into an unsuccessful attempt to dislodge phlegm — and I smiled at what now struck me as adorable quirks. She grunted as she rose to her feet, only marginally taller than me in my sitting position. I bowed my head, and she bestowed upon me the moist, aromatic graces of her phlegm breath, followed by an equally moist gust of breath between my outstretched hands, which I couldn't bring myself to wipe afterward.

She scooted off to my neighbor as I lay down on my back, now fully sober, hands moist. My warped sense of time estimated that the ceremony had at least another hour, and I stared toward the darkness of the ceiling while pondering what to do with my remaining time.

Out of nowhere an enormous blue sky opened above me and then exploded into blinding white like a supernova. The white sheet of sky hurtled toward me, thrust by the infinite weight of the universe crashing down, and within a millisecond it slammed into me, crushing me into countless grains of stardust. Upon impact, a rapturous rush of exhilaration propelled my consciousness forward at hyper speed, leaving behind the scattered infinitesimal pieces of my physical body. A deafening clap reverberated in my ears and in my chest as my consciousness broke through the sheet of light and emerged on the other side, in an unfamiliar realm of humbling enormity. My eyes struggled to focus in the overwhelming light, and immediately after I broke through to the other side, a violent retraction yanked me back into my body as if tethered by a bungee cord.

An adrenaline cocktail of fear and excitement and confusion pumped through me as I gasped through my nostrils. My heart pounded in double time as a frigid shiver ran through my torso and limbs, and I marveled at the late realization that my eyes had been open the whole time.

Without warning, another supernova exploded before my eyes, hurtling a second sheet of blinding white sky that crushed my body with colossal force, smashed out my consciousness and catapulted it forward once more. But this time my consciousness lost momentum and fell shy of breaking through to the other side.

The harrowing flash began and ended within the blink of an eye, but the intensity rattled me to my core, like the combined rush of a lifetime of thrill rides all condensed into a millisecond megadose of adrenaline. I lay breathless on my mat, and the thought of withstanding that intensity for any more than a moment terrified me, but at the same time I knew that tomorrow night I needed to experience of a full dose of Ayahuasca, to see what lies on the other side.

Sharp cramps stabbed at my innards while an enormous bubble of gas bulldozed through my large intestine, and a barrage of Ayahuasca diarrhea followed in its path. The raucous parade of discomfort roared through me as I squirmed in silence, and the next shaman scooted in front of my mat. My intestinal cramping incapacitated me, and by the time I managed to sit up, the shaman had already finished most of her song. My upright position brought a wave of nausea on top of the relentless cramps that still wrenched my innards, and I contorted constantly, unable to focus on her song, unable to sit still as she laid hands and bestowed her breath upon me.

Without a word, she scooted along to my neighbor, and I silently collapsed back down on my mat. As soon as I relaxed, my rectum sounded the alarm of impending diarrhea: an ominous rumbling that implored me to reach a toilet immediately. I had zero confidence that I could contain the storm while shuffling my wobbly legs back and forth, so instead I clenched with all my strength, entwined my legs like a twist tie, and strained for five seconds of eternity until the awful pressure subsided and retreated somewhere back up my large intestine. The diarrhea alarm quieted, but a cacophony of muffled gurgling and high-pitched squeaking erupted from my lower abdomen, reminding me that I had only postponed the inevitable.

The fearsome clutches of Ayahuasca possession loosened, and my closed-eye visuals faded to formless kaleidoscope patterns. They paled in comparison to the lifelike, immersive visions of peak intoxication, but still the illuminated fractals of fluid dancing shapes dazzled me.

One by one the shamans finished their rounds and shuffled back to their mats in the center of the room. Five booming voices faded to four, then three, then two, until only one voice remained: the male shaman sitting in front of my neighbor to the left. The final reverberations of the shaman's song faded, and the background symphony of the jungle transitioned into the foreground. Countless insects, birds, frogs, and unknown creatures filled the silence with a gorgeous interlude of their own song as the shaman scooted his way to the front of my mat. He had begun the ceremony with my neighbor to the right, meaning that I had the honor of receiving a solo serenade for the final performance of the evening. I forced myself to sit upright in full attention as he cleared his throat and eased into a captivating melody that triggered in me a distant, almost forgotten memory of the start of the ceremony, which seemed like years ago.

Though mostly sober, my body still rocked back and forth uncontrollably, swaying in the currents of his song, and I imagined the rest of his audience — the other participants, the other shamans, the jungle creatures — all doing the same. The meaning of his words eluded me, but the aesthetics of the syllables rang out with the beauty of a lyrical masterpiece, and I gave my undivided attention to his song as he poured his heart into it, just as he had done for everyone else.

Upon delivering the final bar of his magnificent melody, he held the last note as an elongated, bittersweet farewell. Blissful gratitude overcame me as I leaned forward and received his breath upon my head and between my outstretched hands. He shuffled back to his position in the center of the room, and everyone waited in silence for some fifteen minutes until the soft voice of a staff member announced the official close of the ceremony.

Even though I knew my hut's bed would be far more comfortable than my thin mat on the stiff wooden floor, I decided to stay put because I barely had the coordination to sit up, and because severe drowsiness and fatigue had already tucked me in for the night. A small parade of more able-bodied participants lumbered toward the door, some of whom seemed entirely sober, while others stomped with clumsy feet that rattled the floorboards beneath my skull.

After the thunderous thumping of feet passed, I closed my eyes and drifted into an unfamiliar state of consciousness, equidistant from the world of dreams, the world of visions, and the waking world. In this dark, dreamless, visionless limbo, I lost track of time but soon heard a soft, high-pitched buzzing, barely perceptible. The buzzing grew exponentially louder as it drew nearer to my ear canal, where it came to an abrupt halt. Something miniscule and nearly weightless landed on my ear.

Terrible memories of that same high-pitched buzzing jolted me awake as I spasmed and swatted at my ear. A lifelong hatred of mosquitoes compelled me to flee to my hut and seek refuge in the sanctuary of my bed's mosquito netting. My previously insurmountable fatigue vanished, and I rushed to gather my pillow and blanket, but a severe lack of balance halted my attempt to stand up. I managed to rise into a seated squat with my buttocks rested on the backs of my heels, and there I remained for several minutes waiting for my equilibrium to recalibrate. I forced another attempt to stand up, but my body refused to cooperate. Wobbly knees exacerbated my lack of balance, and before I could even make it halfway to standing, my buttocks plopped back down to starting position on my heels.

I paused for a moment to recoup, and after taking in several deep breaths, I once again attempted to stand up. Rather than rising in a straight, vertical line, my torso ascended in a shaky zigzag, finally coming to a hunched standing position, so unstable that my mosquito assailant could have toppled me over.

My pillow and blanket provided moral support as I hugged them with both arms, skeptical that the endeavor would end well, but committed to it nonetheless. The darkness of the room blinded me, yet I refrained from illuminating the way, so as not to disturb the nursery of sleeping participants around me. For several long minutes, I stood in place with my upper body wobbling like an ocean buoy, until my subconscious chimed in with some encouragement

"You can do this. You're a big boy."

Dozens of toe-length baby steps carried me to the back wall, which supported my balance and emboldened me to take a whole step all at once, but then a fellow participant shattered my concentration as he strutted past at normal walking speed. Compared to my snail's pace, he blew past me like a racehorse, throwing me into a dizzy loss of balance, and I grasped at the wall to keep from tumbling over. What should have been a ten-second stroll turned into a harrowing ten-minute odyssey, but I managed to reach the exit where I spent several more minutes wrestling with the door until I remembered that it opened inward, not outward.

Halfway through my slow journey down the stairs, the door behind me flew open, and another able-bodied participant trotted toward me. I cowered in fear at the sound of her steady, confident feet, and I prayed that she wouldn't talk to me, because I needed to devote all my mental effort toward not falling down the steps. I hugged the railing like a frightened koala, and after she scurried off into the shadows of the jungle, I started breathing again.

Some sixty seconds later, I conquered the few remaining stairs and then somehow managed to put on my shoes. As I stumbled through the dark, narrow, uneven, unfamiliar dirt paths of the jungle, each clumsy step sobered me little by little. Only a few minutes into the journey, my pace doubled, rivaling that of an energetic senior citizen.

I arrived at my hut ahead of schedule, clomped up the small flight of wooden stairs, shed my clothing, and then crashed headfirst into bed, failing to appreciate that the diarrhea emergency of moments ago had mysteriously disappeared. Disjointed and unintelligible fragments of misfiring thoughts ricocheted in my mind for several minutes until suddenly the clamor crashed to a halt, and in pristine silence a booming question lassoed my attention. It came to me from parts unknown, in my own voice, addressed from myself to myself.

"Why do I hate mosquitoes so much?"

In the same instant that I comprehended the question, the answer flashed through my mind.

"The camping trip."

The answer referred to a long-forgotten family camping trip during my youth, where a swarm of mosquitoes infiltrated our tent and waited in ambush until nighttime when we sealed ourselves inside. I spent the first several hours of that night swatting at the faint, high-pitched buzzing sounds in my ears while mosquitoes elsewhere on my body gorged themselves on the all-you-can-eat buffet of my young blood. I spent the next hour of that night trying to keep my head tucked inside the safe but sweltering refuge of my sleeping bag, coming up for air every few minutes, only to be bitten again. I fled from the tent and relocated to the fortress of our family minivan, but it sealed in the nighttime summer heat and roasted me like an oven. When I made the mistake of cracking open a window, a new legion of mosquitoes snuck in and devoured me. They indulged in a gluttonous feast, evidenced by the dozens of itchy, red welts that covered my body the next morning.

As I reflected on that camping trip, the sudden sound of heavy feet on wooden steps startled my train of thought off its rails. The residual effects of Ayahuasca still slightly skewed my sense of hearing, and I couldn't discern where the sounds originated — perhaps just my neighbor walking up his steps, or perhaps some lost soul stumbling up my steps by mistake. Paranoia seeped in, and I imagined the intruder must be the same fast-trotting woman who had frightened me on the stairs of the ceremonial hut, that she had gone down the wrong jungle path in an Ayahuasca daze, gotten lost, and had now come back to haunt me again.

Two streams of independent thought babbled back and forth at each other without any conscious input from me.

"Just say 'I believe you have the wrong hut' and she'll go away."

"No, that could be confusing."

"Why's that?"

"Because you need to get her attention first. She won't know who you're talking to."

"True."

53

Unlike a typical dialogue where two speakers take turns speaking, and where one word logically follows another, in this dialogue every word from both sides of the entire conversation all flashed through my mind at once. The dialogue ended in the same instant that it began. After a short deliberation, I concluded that opening with a simple, inquisitive "Hello?" would be best.

I rose to my forearms and turned my head toward the door, then sighed in relief upon realizing that the sound originated from my neighbor's hut. My mind eased for the first time in what felt like hours, no longer concerned with threats of bedroom intruders, or mosquito attacks, or falling down steps. My weary head crashed face-first into my pillow, and my thoughts turned to the Ayahuasca visions still fresh in memory.

I pondered my confusing sexual encounter with the Urchin Queen, which I had initially written off as a bizarre merger of my elevated libido and my fear of the porcupine tree. But upon further consideration, I realized that the Urchin Queen represented a different type of fear — one that I had unknowingly harbored, and one that I would spend many more nights thinking about: the fear of intimacy.

Second Night with Ayahuasca

The brightness of the morning sun penetrated my closed eyelids deep enough to reach my slumbering consciousness. My eyes parted open, a sliver just wide enough to confirm that I was indeed in the Amazon, and that I hadn't lost my mind. Contrary to most mornings, not a trace of any dreams remained in memory, as if I had awoken from a seven-hour blackout.

A residual fear of toppling over still lingered as I rose to my feet, but aside from minor lightheadedness and dehydration, I suffered no discernible hangover. To the contrary, blissful serenity permeated my mind, I felt rejuvenated, and I smiled as my sturdy legs walked me to the bathroom.

The toilet consisted of a large plastic bucket affixed inside of a knee-height wooden box with a flimsy plastic Western toilet seat screwed onto the top. Despite the wretched gurgling noises that haunted my intestines the previous night, out from my rear came not the anticipated sloshy mess of raging diarrhea, but a firm, healthy bowel movement, unremarkable except for a strange foreign odor, the likes of which I had never produced before.

After burying my fecal matter using the provided sawdust, I washed my hands at the makeshift sink: a bucket of water and a scooping bowl that sat next to a sagging porcelain basin jerry-rigged into the wooden bathroom wall and attached to a drainage pipe. I then suited up in my long-sleeve pajama armor and strode out the door, toward the dining hall for breakfast.

The tropical sun and the beautiful sights and sounds of the surrounding jungle amplified the unexpected tranquility that flowed through me. Only twenty-four hours prior, the same sun, the same jungle, the same sights and sounds had merely been a welcome reprieve from city life, but the afterglow of Ayahuasca intoxication transformed my surroundings into an invigorating paradise that electrified me, and I felt ecstatic simply to be alive.

In the dining hall a man and a woman discussed their experiences from the previous night. She seemed intelligent and she spoke English as her native language, but her inarticulate descriptions painted only a blurry picture of vague concepts, exacerbated by her chronic habit of adding the -y suffix to words in order to make them adjective-y.

Sitting across the table, her one-man audience listened with engaged, focused eyes. He spoke English as a second language, with a thick accent but excellent grammar and vocabulary. His replies occasionally started with long gaps of silence as he appeared to scan his vast lexicon for the precise words that he desired. A courteous gentleman, he listened with sincere interest as the woman across from him struggled to construct a full sentence.

"And it was, like...flashbacky, and, like...oh, I don't know. I can't really describe it. Anyway, how was your experience?"

His eyes widened and his head bobbed up and down in a slow, seemingly involuntary nod. He prefaced his response with a long hesitation, as if not only searching for adequate wording but also deep in reflection of a profound experience.

"I..."

His eyes remained fixed on a distant focal point as his head continued bobbing up and down.

"I deedn't may-kit to za toy-let..."

She confided that she also had a close call, narrowly making it to the bathroom in time, and their confessions provided solace in knowing that if I soiled myself mid-ceremony, I would be neither the first nor probably the last.

At the buffet I gathered onto my plate some fresh fruit and some unidentifiable gruel that resembled oatmeal, along with a tall glass of freshly squeezed passion fruit juice. I spotted a table with vacancy, and upon approaching I made eye contact with a middle-aged man who sat listening to the simultaneous conversations crisscrossing over each other along the table. He and I exchanged a cordial smile and a nod as I motioned toward the empty, plastic lawn chair beside him.

"Is this seat taken?"

"We were saving it for you!"

I widened my smile and settled into my spot, nodding at a few additional neighbors who extended casual greetings amid the crossfire of conversations.

The fresh and all-natural food on my plate looked delectable, but putting it in my mouth, chewing it, and swallowing it, all felt like laborious chores. Despite my complete lack of appetite, I force-fed myself each bite, motivated only by the gaping nineteen hours since my last meal.

By lunchtime my regular appetite returned, allowing me to fully appreciate the buffet of scrumptious delights — wholesome, real foods, straight from the earth, prepared not by the cold steel hands of assembly line robots, but by the warm loving hands of someone I could thank in person. I savored a heaping plateful and considered going back for seconds, but then nixed that idea for fear of how the digested food would exit my body. Thus far I had avoided the wrath of Ayahuasca diarrhea and vomiting, and I feared supplying excess munitions for either.

The dining hall still clamored with activity as I retired to my hut for an afternoon nap in the jungle's oppressive daytime humidity. Perhaps an hour later, I awoke exactly as I had fallen asleep — sweaty and disgusting — and though a cold floral bath sounded splendid, I fought the temptation and vowed to be sweaty and disgusting for a week, rather than once again risk a typhoid infection through the open wounds on my feet.

I spent the rest of the day in a mixed state of contemplation, excitement, and mild anxiety about my first full dose. My face puckered up at the thought of the taste, and I hoped that the bitter onslaught would be easier to swallow the second time around.

But come nightfall, the acrid brew dashed those hopes as soon as it touched my lips, somehow tasting more awful than the previous night, and double the size of my previous dose. It required two strenuous gulps for me to force it down, and then also required a diligent effort to keep it down. Nausea and lightheadedness struck within seconds, and I tiptoed back to my mat to await blast off. After the last participant returned to his mat, the staff extinguished the lanterns, darkness overtook the room, and within fifteen minutes the effects trickled in.

The myriad sounds of the jungle unpegged themselves from their stationary positions and swirled around me in a surreal medley of spiraling surround sound. I sat in the epicenter of a sonorous whirlpool of croaking, hooting, howling, chirping, and clicking that poured into the funnels of my ears.

A cocktail of natural scents and man-made aromas titillated the depths of my nostrils. An eclectic amalgam of soil, plant life, the nearby stream, my own body scent, my neighbor's tobacco, and the musk of an approaching rainstorm merged into a symbiotic, aromatic blend in which each scent complemented the others without sacrificing its own individuality.

An immense yawn brewed in my throat like a delayed sneeze, tingling with exotic energy. It expanded throughout my chest, slowly bubbled up the back of my throat, and then stopped behind my ears. With a sudden and uncontainable force, it exploded outward as my mouth thrust itself open to an alarming width, like a serpent dislocating its jaw before feeding. Every muscle from my chest upward strained with quivering intensity, and a tremendous inhale stifled my hearing, lasting for what felt like minutes as my face attempted to eat itself.

Amicable fatigue laid a soft hand upon my shoulder, encouraged me with a gentle nudge to relax, and then guided my head down to my pillow. As I snuggled into position, the smooth sound of my rustling hair pacified me, and the soft valley of the pillow embraced me like a glorious scalp massage. My torso relaxed and my legs extended, melting away all anxiety and tension, and my lungs filled with a delicious breath of cool jungle air that sedated me.

The songs of the shamans faded in and took hold of me, first prompting my foot to fidget, then prompting my jaw to wiggle from side to side, forcing my teeth to tap-dance inside my mouth. My involuntary movements escalated with the intensity of the singing shamans, and a wild fidgeting crawled up my right leg, spreading like contagious laughter. It then spread to my left leg and electrified my lower half with a warm, uncontainable energy that further spread to my arms and hands. My restless limbs demanded constant readjusting and repositioning, and if I had the coordination to stand up, I might have defied my lifelong aversion to dancing. But a sudden loss of motor skill confined me to lying on my mat, where I tossed and turned in silence as the first shaman circled around to me.

Despite the hyperactivity coursing through my limbs and jaw, severe fatigue dominated my body and prohibited me from even sitting up. I mustered only a half sit-up before collapsing back to my mat and offering a silent, stuttering apology to the shaman as he began his song.

Soft syllables of the Shipibo language streamed from his lips to my ears in an undulating wave, swimming like a sea snake and taking possession of me as it penetrated my ears.

My lips trembled, brimming with the urge to vocalize something. They joined in the uncontrollable movements of my jaw, and the two danced together as I silently spoke in tongues. The shaman belted out the crescendo of his song, and my lips and tongue flailed, spewing an inaudible barrage of syllables. I struggled to read my uncontrollable lips, but I gleaned only that the syllables didn't resemble any language familiar to me. As an emphatic punctuation to each unintelligible verse, my tongue shot straight out of my mouth, fully extended, and then flicked up and down like a serpent in search of food.

Beginning in my fingertips, the warm currents of hyperactive energy transformed into a cold, tingling numbness that crept into my hands. Pins and needles marched up my forearms and held their ground at my elbows, harassing me with chilly, low voltage currents that pulsed through each funny bone. At the same time, a harsh cramping pinched at my innards, worse than the night before and accompanied by equally unpleasant bloating. My underwear's elastic waistband constricted my abdomen and exacerbated my discomfort as tremendous gas bubbles stormed through me, so with my cold, numb fingers, I propped up the waistband off my abdomen to allow minor reprieve.

The phrase "this hurts" echoed in my mind, followed by a realization that I couldn't determine the tense of my own two-word sentence, that I couldn't comprehend the concepts of past, present, and future, and that all three had melted away into a cauldron of murky thoughts and imagery stripped of their timestamps. Memories of the past masqueraded as present experiences. Present experiences masqueraded as future premonitions. Thoughts of the future masqueraded as memories of the past.

Before my mind's eye, a diagram of my temporal distortion manifested into a triangular emblem that resembled the recycling symbol. Three folded arrows represented the trifecta of past, present, and future, each arrow pointing toward its neighbor — past to present, present to future, future to past — forming an infinite, triangular loop. I failed to understand the emblem overlaid upon the flashing visions, and it only disoriented me further.

Amidst the noise of my ensuing mental confusion, a low-pitched mechanical humming like that of an oil tanker rumbled in the far reaches of my mind, and although a tremendous distance away, the heavy bass of the vibrations rattled my skull as the deafening wall of humming approached.

From across the room, over the songs of the shamans and the thunderous humming in my head, a woman repeatedly moaned in ecstasy, distracting me for a moment until the humming drowned out everything in the physical world.

In a slow ascent from my mat, I floated out of my body and hovered an arm's length above myself, looking down into my closed eyes. The deafening hum faded to silence as I watched myself squirm in pain from the cramping and bloating, and I watched my body repeatedly spasm as it clenched to prevent soiling itself. My detached consciousness felt no pain, but through a frail line of communication to my writhing body, the gastrointestinal discomfort and the strenuous energy of clenched muscles resonated in me like seismic waves.

As if convulsing awake from a nightmare, my consciousness crashed back into my clenched body, lassoed back into the physical world by the wretched clamor of what sounded like a fatal vomiting. The victim sat a mere two mats away as he strained and heaved in a futile attempt to expel his innards, and my heightened sense of hearing swallowed up in vivid detail every gurgle, every dilation and contraction of his esophagus, and every multilayered choking spasm. I expected to start dry heaving myself, but just like on the previous night, uncontrollable laughter ambushed me, forcing me to bite down on my lips as my chest heaved. Rolling onto my side facing away from him helped me to refocus and turn my attention inward.

I instantly teleported to the world of visions, lying naked on my back, alone in the soft billowing blankets of a heavenly bed. Though I didn't recognize my surroundings, the warmth of the bed suggested that I had been lying there for some time. My back nestled into the soothing texture of the fabrics that held long-preserved reservoirs of body heat, and the surrounding mountain range of cool fabrics collapsed and folded against my skin as I sprawled out. The bed's realism surpassed that of the uncomfortable mat from whence I had come, and my limbs quivered in delight as I stretched out like a yawning feline.

My hands rose into view, and instead of the scruffy male fingers of my familiar Caucasian hands, I wielded two petite, elegant, unfamiliar hands of darker complexion, with slender, feminine fingers and glossy well-kept fingernails. My own identity baffled me, and I whipped my head around in search of a mirror, but darkness shrouded my surroundings.

My ladylike fingers took on a mind of their own, skating a figure eight along my abdomen, skimming the surface of my unfamiliar body. My feminine skin — soft and hairless and free of blemishes — radiated with an arousing, healthy vibrancy. The meandering fingers of my right hand navigated south on the foreign terrain and arrived between my legs to find no sign of manhood, but rather a smooth, bald patch surrounding two folds of soft flesh lightly clinging to each other, with a hint of moisture seeping out from between them. My fingertips grazed and tickled the protruding perimeter, drawing slow circles around the delicate folds and painting them with a light glaze of their own moisture, then parting them to expose the warm entrance of a sleek and narrow opening.

My palm rested just above the bare opening while my fingers caressed and teased the parted lips for what felt like an eternity, until my middle and ring fingers curled back inward and delved into the warmth of my body. Silky lubrication coated my fingers as they slid in knuckle-deep, and I gasped at the realism of my snug body warmth hugging my fingers.

My lower abdomen faded to transparency, mimicking the Urchin Queen, to whom I had made gruesome love the previous night. I strained my neck in a half sit-up and peered through my flexed abdomen's clear layers to see a soft glow of white and orange sunburst radiating outward from my opening. Normally hidden from sight, the mysterious internal walls of self-lubricating flesh entranced me with their sleekness and dazzled me with their perfectly accommodating elasticity, and I trembled as my amplified sense of touch bombarded me with every fine detail of the warm canal's smooth texture. My entire body throbbed with swelling arousal, and despite my gasping I couldn't catch my breath.

A sharp, cramping pain stabbed at my intestines and yanked me from the vision, and I squirmed on my mat while wincing with a sour face. A massive cloud of malevolent gas shoved its way through me, and a thunderous gurgling boomed from somewhere north of my rectum, fully audible over the five singing shamans.

I shifted my attention away from the pain and toward the voices of the shamans, but their individual locations eluded me: their songs all merged into a voluminous amalgamation of liquid sound pouring into my ears. The severity of my disorientation had likewise eluded me: I realized that several of the shamans may have already passed me, and that I could not recall any of my introspective intentions.

Involuntary mental spasms obfuscated my thinking and hindered my concentration, as if a swindler repeatedly concealed and shuffled my thoughts in an unwinnable game of mental Three-card Monte. At the same time, autonomous and independent trains of thought liberally leapt from one set of tracks to another. Helplessness sank in as I lost the ability to focus or formulate a complete thought, and my desperate grip on sanity slowly slipped away.

Sleeves of pins and needles constricted my arms. A tempest of diarrhea repeatedly slammed like a battering ram against the wall of my clenched sphincter and required all the strength in my body to prevent a putrid mess. Upon my brow, accumulated sweat rolled toward my eyes, but wiping my numb hands across my forehead merely smeared more perspiration, and a layer of profuse sweat covered my entire body.

Exhaustion, tingles, and my haywire train of thought all competed to bully me further into shambles, and I trembled in terror at the thought of enduring the overwhelming intensity not only for a few more hours, but for five more ceremonies. The thought petrified me at my animal core, like encountering a wild predator face-to-face, looking into its bloodthirsty eyes and collapsing under the weight of hopelessness. Incapable of words or thoughts, my mind abandoned hope and flooded itself with the adrenaline of utmost terror.

Over the spiraling sound of the shamans and the jungle creatures, a rumbling of thunder foretold the impending arrival of a rainstorm that brewed in the distance. The momentary distraction graced me with a brief moment of mental clarity, and my subconscious gathered the strength to throw a lifeline in the form of two simple words.

"Everything passes."

I latched on to the words like a castaway, mentally clinging to the only life jacket in an ocean of chaos. My disheveled wreck of a body mustered enough mental and physical coordination to whisper the words back to myself, and they resonated with irrefutable truth: that my mental disorientation, the numbness and tingling in my limbs, the profuse sweating, the cramping pain and gastrointestinal distress — everything would eventually end, no matter how intense, no matter how unpleasant, and I basked in the salvation of their impermanence. Long, deep breaths filled my lungs and helped me regain composure.

The nourishment of the crisp jungle air flowed into my lungs and then spread outward to my extremities, infusing me with serenity and relief. Each subsequent breath further infused me with buoyant bliss that elevated me out of the blackened depths of despair.

Upon my chest, the weight and warmth of my sweaty folded arms comforted me, like the reassuring touch of a loved one. An irresistible urge to hug myself overwhelmed me, so I wrapped my arms around my shoulders, embracing my torso as it heaved with each deep breath.

The humid smell of rain wafted into my nostrils while a flash of lightning illuminated the hut's interior and reintroduced me to my long-forgotten surroundings. A stampede of rolling thunder marched across the sky and vibrated in my chest, and my sense of hearing slowly recovered from its dementia. The spiraling, jumbled mess of indistinguishable noises unfurled into five distinct songs of the shamans. Beauty poured into my ears from the male shaman two positions to my left, and a light rain merged into the symphony with graceful power, crashing upon the hut's thatched roof and the jungle canopy.

Though I had writhed in a sticky coat of sweat only moments before, the temperature in the hut plummeted as the storm's cool breeze caressed my sweaty face and encouraged me to snuggle under my blanket. I obliged with giddy eagerness, tucking myself in chin deep, and then rewrapping my arms around myself underneath the blanket. My body heat and the pleasant chill of the breeze complemented each other, and my enthusiastic hug amplified the intensity of both.

Jungle aromas mixed with that of the rain and filled my lungs with breath after breath of uncanny rejuvenation and bliss, each more invigorating than the last. An explosion of butterflies in my stomach tickled me with nearly unbearable excitement as I floated on clouds of ecstasy. My heart pounded in my chest, the feverish contractions pumping euphoria throughout my body, while my eyes clenched and wrung out unexpected tears of joy that rolled down my cheeks.

A roaring whoosh muffled the sounds of the ceremony, and my stomach dropped as I plummeted in darkness into the unfathomable depths of my mind, until slamming into the floor of my subconscious. The fierce and disorienting impact obliterated my sense of self, leaving me dazed and confused, surrounded by darkness, unsure of my identity, but sure that I wasn't Nicholas.

My blurry vision slowly faded into focus, and from the perspective of my ex-girlfriend I found myself lying naked in bed, on my back, with my smooth, hairless legs in the air. My boyfriend, Nicholas, thrust inside me as he hoisted my lower half into the air, forming a sling with his arms and gripping the cheeks of my rear with two firm hands. Our carnal desires spilled out in irrepressible moans, reciprocally amplifying the sexual energy that surged between us, and our slick bodies glistened with the sweat of passionate vigor. I traced my delicate fingers down his abdomen as my legs grabbed hold of his waist and pulled him closer into me. I begged with my eyes for stronger thrusting, he obliged with a grin, and the sound of our wet flesh slapping together rivaled the volume of my emphatic moaning.

The warmth of his bare flesh melded into mine as he effortlessly glided in and out of me, and my arousal soared as I watched him revel in undiluted pleasure. Animal lust intoxicated him as he clenched his eyes and parted his mouth open with intensified panting. He strained his sweaty face, and the veins in his neck bulged. He gnashed his teeth and then bit his bottom lip while struggling to postpone his impending climax. He tightened his grip on my rear, and I tightened my legs around his waist as I arched my back. I felt him swelling inside me, on the brink of erupting with explosive bursts. I salivated with lust, yearning for his seed, and I prayed that this would be the time that he finally threw caution to the wind and finished inside me.

But he opened his eyes, released his bite on his bottom lip, slowed his thrust to a halt, and then withdrew himself from me without a grand finale, or a finale of any kind. He scooted back and reached across the bed, into his desk drawer, and though he was still close enough to touch, he now felt eternally distant. Over the soft sound of the crinkling wrapper in his hands, he reluctantly muttered half to me and half to himself.

"I should prolly use one of these..."

The cold and lifeless latex in his hand matched the cold and lifeless mood of the room. He looked me in the eye and offered an apologetic smile, sincere but ineffective. I feigned a smile in return, disguising my heartbreak and disappointment. I knew that he cared about me, but feelings of inadequacy crept in and taunted me, sneering that I wasn't good enough for him.

He faded away into the black background, leaving me all alone. My throat tightened up, my chest ached, and I shivered as a spine-chilling sense of inferiority tormented me. In a flailing free fall from the upper echelon of sexual pleasure, I plummeted to the cold, hard tundra of heartbreak, smashing face first into the surface. Like the viscous yellow guts of a squished maggot, my unfulfilled desire splattered out from the force of impact, leaving me with a mangled sack of lacerated flesh and broken bones. I wallowed in painful self-pity, and I closed my eyes in a vain attempt to contain my tears.

My eyes remained clenched shut as I returned to my physical body lying motionless on my mat. Palpable, dreadful feelings of inadequacy and self-pity festered inside me, eroding away my self-esteem and sense of worth. I tried to swallow but gagged instead. My throat ached and quivered as it tightened, constricted by the brutal grip of melancholy.

My conscience waited to let the oppressive emotions fully sink in, and then it whispered to me in a calm voice.

"Now you know how she felt."

My insulted ego hurled a defensive, knee-jerk objection and attempted to sidestep the point.

"Da hell outta here! What, was I just supposed to knock her up!? I had to use protection! It was the responsible thing to do!"

Not fooled by my ego's semantic sleight of hand, my conscience replied in the same calm voice.

"And now you know how she felt."

My ego huffed and puffed and wrung its hands in a desperate search for a retort, but came up dry, and then stomped off with bursts of aggravated exhales. A long, painful silence followed, forcing me to think about it from her perspective, and forcing me to concede my own selfishness — that I never should have put her in that position in the first place.

I opened my eyes, and though I couldn't see anything in the darkness, I patted myself down to confirm that I was still Nicholas, that I still had furry man-paws and male genitalia, and that I still rested on an uncomfortable mat in a thatched-roof hut in the Amazon rainforest. But the weight of severe intoxication pressed my eyes shut and instantly forced me back into the world of visions.

Utter darkness surrounded me as I wandered, lost and confused, unable to discern if I was enclosed by black walls or simply looking off into empty infinity. I turned my head to the side, looking for an entrance or an exit or anything at all, but found only darkness. As I turned my head back, my peripheral vision caught the glowing, menacing eyes of a shadowy beast — two yellow embers in a blur of white and gray fur charging at me in stealthy silence. Before I could even react, a deranged canine lunged at me with slobbering jaws and sank his fangs into my arm.

The adrenaline of the attack stood his thick coat of gray fur on end, firm like bristles, as he clamped down his powerful jaws like a bear trap, grinding his teeth against my bone, securing an inescapable death lock. He whipped his head back and forth, his teeth and fangs ripping the flesh from my arm, and he gurgled on a mixture of blood and saliva that shot outward with his ferocious growling.

Natural instincts seized me, and I dug my heels into the ground, nearly losing balance as I pulled back with all my strength. I jerked my arm back, further ripping my flesh and muscle as the canine's clamped jaws scraped down the length of my forearm, his teeth etching jagged grooves into my bones. I recoiled in horror, but his jaws clamped tighter the more I pulled back. For a split second, a transparent image of a Chinese finger trap flickered before my eyes and hinted at the futility of my resistance, a hint that initially eluded me in the throes of the terrifying struggle, but which struck me moments later. My whirling panic crashed to a halt as I narrowed my eyes and realized that giving in was the only way out.

In the same instant that I relaxed and stopped resisting, the bloodthirsty canine released his grip on my arm and ceased his growling. Soothing hues of baby blue extinguished the fire in his fearsome eyes, and his fur softened and fell flat. He extended his long, wet tongue and playfully wiped my shredded flesh from his lips as the bloody scraps fell to his feet.

He took two courteous steps back to give us space, and then he sat with perfect posture like a well-trained household pet, ears pricked in attention, awaiting my command. With an open palm I extended my mangled arm toward him, offering my dangling flesh as a meal, and my exposed bone as a chew toy. But in a proud display of impeccable manners, he sat unflinching, looking up at me with wide, unblinking eyes, head cocked at a slight angle, still awaiting my command.

We stared at each other for a moment before I broke the silence with the first question that struck me:

"Who are you?"

Thousands of faces flashed before me in a dizzying high-speed montage, like a slot machine rotating through the portraits of every person I had ever known. The spinning blur of portraits gradually slowed, intermittently pausing to show ex-bosses, friends, ex-girlfriends, and relatives, living and deceased; then, with a loud and final click, the montage disappeared as the patient, well-behaved canine transformed into my father. We stood face-to-face, looking into each other's eyes without a word, and before I could formulate a response, he faded away into the backdrop of eternal darkness.

The vision slipped from my mental grasp, and my desperate attempts to re-immerse myself proved futile. I toiled over the meaning of the vision and its abrupt ending, but it left me so confused that I wondered if it had any meaning at all.

My deep concentration distracted me from realizing that the shamans had finished their rounds long ago, that the room had fallen silent other than the soft serenade of the jungle, and that I had lost all sense of time.

I suddenly found myself sitting at the wooden desk in my hut, blank journal pages in front of me, pen in hand, Ayahuasca visions slowly fading from memory. A foreign stream of consciousness mumbled antsy imperatives at me.

"C'mon, hurry up'n write it down. Gotta write this all down before you forget."

I pressed my pen against the blank page, and my point of view zoomed in to a microscopic level, as if seen from the perspective of a flea on the page. The towering pen's ballpoint tip etched millimeter-wide canyons as it rolled across the vast plateau of paper dampened by jungle humidity. Rivers of black ink flooded into the freshly carved canyons — the smooth lines and curves of elegant but indecipherable glyphs. My vision panned out for a full view of the page, and the foreign symbols danced in a perpetual metamorphosis from one character to another, like the fluid, shape-shifting text sometimes seen in dreamland.

The exotic symbols resembled a hybrid of English and Japanese calligraphy, but they exuded a uniqueness that confounded me. The longer I stared at them the less they made sense, and the notion of written language itself began to lose meaning. It struck me as preposterous that arbitrary scribbles could convey thoughts, and I scoffed at the idea of an alphabet, of written language, of putting pen to paper for any reason. Equally incredulous became the notion of spoken language, and my mind discarded the use of words altogether, reverting to a primordial consciousness consisting of only raw emotions. Silent, wordless feelings of disbelief wracked my mind as I gazed down at the page of glyphs and refused to accept the concept of language. Under the weight of their own absurdity, the black strokes of ink shattered like fallen Christmas ornaments, bursting apart and splintering into trails of microscopic dust that snaked across the page until a gust of my scoffing breath whisked away the preposterous contaminants.

From the center of the hut, a quiet voice wafted into my ears, barely audible to me as I floated in the world of visions.

"Good evening, everyone. The ceremony is now closed."

My consciousness rejoined my body and locked back into place behind my eyes, but my body still felt foreign, inorganic, and mechanical, like a robotic transportation vehicle that my consciousness operated via remote control. My repeated attempts to send the command "sit up straight" mostly failed to register, while the few that did register resulted in only a short fit of twitching, strained abdominals, and quiet mumbling of the word *diarrhea*.

A shadowy figure from across the room clicked on her flashlight, and the unrestrained light flooded the hut with blinding rays of white. My jittery eyes squinted in a hopeless attempt to identify the perpetrator, and I watched in envy as her anonymous silhouette scampered out of the exit, home free and toilet bound.

Her swift mobility inspired my robot body — the vehicle on which I depended — to likewise head for the exit. In small, gradual steps of piecemeal resurrection, the vehicle remembered how to function, first clasping its hands open and closed, then rotating its shoulders in small shrugs, then stretching out both legs, and then bending both knees to signal "all systems go". Without any direct input from my consciousness, the vehicle autonomously leaned to its side and gathered our bedding supplies in preparation for the journey.

I gave the command to rise, and after a three-second delay the vehicle complied in small increments, first rising to its knees, then to a seated squat — one foot at a time while balancing on its knuckles like a gorilla — and then, over the course of ten seconds, to a wobbly but vertical standing position. We limped our way one baby step at a time toward the sturdy back wall — our savior and guarantor of balance, our guiding beacon that led us safely to the exit in the dark.

Rough and haphazard patches of insect screen protruded from all edges of the door and gently scraped against the wooden frame as my robot body drew open the door. The dark staircase daunted us both, and I instructed the vehicle to test the waters of each step using its big toe first before committing any weight. The vehicle complied, clutching the handrail and progressing one slow step at a time, in a harrowing descent that sobered us both, repairing our disconnection and unifying us again into a single being.

At the bottom of the steps, I located my shoes and put them on with ease, which instilled a false sense of confidence in my motor skills, and within my first few steps I nearly tumbled to the ground as my legs attempted to walk away from each other. Though my consciousness and physical body had reunited, each step home still required the balance and concentration of a tightrope walker, forcing me to disregard the bloodcurdling cries and moans that tore through the jungle as a distant neighbor expelled his stomach contents.

My slow march through the jungle drew me closer to home, and the thought of lying down in my bed filled me with delight, but my heart sank when I looked up to see a fellow participant marching toward me, his balance far exceeding my own. I had no desire to converse and no confidence in my ability to do so, and for a moment I considered retreating down a different path, but getting lost in the jungle frightened me more than the ordeal of human interaction.

From a few paces away he recognized me and blurted out an immediate salutation.

"Hey there!"

His simple, two-word greeting resounded with eloquence compared to my grunt of a reply with squinted eyes and an oafish smile.

At his silent insistence, we embraced with a long and drawn-out hug. We had only met two days prior and had barely exchanged words since then, which tainted the embrace with a hint of awkwardness, but I appreciated the gesture nonetheless. He released his grip, but my shaky hands clung to his shoulders, and I realized too late that he misconstrued my prolonged contact as deep brotherly love, when I had only intended to secure my wobbly balance.

In a sober state of mind, I would have been happy to chat, but in my current state of mind, even simple conversation felt agonizing and impossible. I prayed that he would bid me an abrupt farewell, and that I could simply nod and retreat to my bed, but he dashed my hopes with the last thing that I wanted to hear: a question.

"So how was your experience?"

None of the right words came to me, and after a long, awkward silence, a vague and clumsy response dribbled out of my mouth.

"Mmm...it...was...uh...good?"

My ineptitude filled me with embarrassment, and I followed up with an equally slow-witted apology.

"Sorry...still kinda...scatterbrained."

He smiled and shrugged it off, insisting that it was nothing to apologize for. I hoped that he would pick up on my blatant inability to converse, and that he would end our interaction, but to my dismay he launched into a zealous recount of his own experience, none of which made sense to me. My focus faded, and a sudden lightheadedness carried me away from the conversation.

My consciousness floated out of my skull, leaving the vehicle of my robot body unattended and reeling from the barrage of unintelligible words that bounced off its forehead and challenged its already questionable balance.

He left me no choice but to interrupt his monologue, so I butted in with a loud and awkward hum, followed by a sloppy slur of a farewell.

"MMMmmm...arrright...catch you...to-...morrow."

He chuckled, we embraced once more, and I hoped that he would forgive my manners.

I stumbled my way back to my hut, up the front stairs and straight to the toilet. My bare hind parts plopped down upon the flimsy plastic throne, and I anticipated an unruly mess of diarrhea, as prophesized by my ominous gastrointestinal rumblings during the ceremony. But once again my bowel movement surprised me with its banality, unremarkable except for the accompanying plume of hideous gas.

I had pondered in advance the conundrum of how best to wipe my rear in the dark of night with no electricity. Using the paltry illumination of my ancient dumbphone seemed problematic for multiple reasons: losing one hand to hold the phone, having to press a key every ten seconds to keep the screen illuminated, the risk of dropping my phone in the toilet, etc. However, this seemed preferable over using the hut's kerosene lantern, which I envisioned my inebriated self accidentally knocking over, starting a fire in the cramped bathroom during my most vulnerable moment, with my feet shackled by the underwear around my ankles, and with a mess upon my rear. So I opted for the juggling act of balancing my phone in one hand while wiping myself with the other.

After the first wipe, I shined my phone upon the used toilet paper to reveal a bathroom miracle, the bowel movement equivalent to a gymnast's perfect ten: a turd of perfect consistency that left no visible trace on the toilet paper. The revelation dumbfounded and delighted me as I pulled up my underwear, sprinkled some sawdust, washed my hands at the sink, and then stumbled to bed.

As I collapsed into bed, my right hand fell to the inside of my thigh, resting beside my groin. Even with my ecstatic mind free of lewd thoughts, the mere presence of my hand excited my attention-starved genitals. An unstoppable flow of blood rushed to the scene and inflated my member, pinning it against my thigh, trapped there by my underpants, bent at an uncomfortable angle that demanded remediation.

I reached down my underpants to straighten the kinked hose and let my unsolicited engorgement subside, fully intent on respecting the rules of the retreat. The warmth of my hand and the sensation of flesh on flesh caught me off guard, and a heavy jolt of repressed pleasure coursed through my body, teasing me like a naughty lover as I rushed to adjust myself into a neutral position.

My erection swelled to full engorgement, throbbing with unwanted sexual energy, weighing heavy upon my lower abdomen and pulsating to the rhythm of my heartbeat. It refused to subside, and the stubborn erection prophesized a dire omen of repressed carnal desires determined to haunt me throughout the retreat and distract me from meaningful introspection. A weary sigh deflated my lungs but not my member as the reality sank in — that unsolicited erections and lewd visions would only increase with time — and for a moment I contemplated the only viable solution: breaking the rules of the retreat, and exorcising the demon.

First Day of Rest

An air of nervous hesitance hung about the room as the twenty of us sat in a large circle awaiting the commencement of our first group sharing session. We all glanced around the room at each other, flashing forced smiles upon accidental eye contact, and no one appeared eager to share. We had only met each other a few days prior, and most of us had exchanged words with only a few other participants, so we were mostly still strangers to each other.

Our facilitator sat at the circle's twelve o'clock position, deliberating out loud to herself whether to start the sharing in a clockwise or counterclockwise rotation. The two adjacent participants to her left and to her right fidgeted with uneasy hope that the rotation would start away from them and spare them the awful fate of being first.

Sitting near the six o'clock position afforded me a luxury of time to mull over which of my experiences to share, and which ones to discard into the pile of unmentionables. But my luxury of prep time felt grossly inadequate for the monumental task at hand: trying to compress two nights of Ayahuasca visions into a coherent five-minute summary.

Simply being able to remember the visions presented a challenge. Much like dreams, the visions raced to disappear from memory, but I had managed to hang on to them long enough to document them in my journal, perhaps thanks to my longtime pursuit of lucid dreaming, and my many hours devoted to strengthening my dream recall. However, having less than forty-eight hours to reflect on the first ceremony, and less than twenty-four hours to reflect on the second, trying to narrate the confounding visions presented another challenge altogether, exacerbated by their subjective and personal nature.

Our facilitator motioned counterclockwise, toward her right-hand side.

"Let's start this way, shall we?"

The unlucky participant to the right rolled her eyes and slouched with an exaggerated expression of hopeless defeat, while the lucky participant to the left smiled and discharged an audible sigh of relief.

One by one, we shared our experiences as best we could while the group listened in silent, focused attention. Some participants struggled to clear even the first hurdle of remembering their visions. Some participants cleared the first hurdle with vivid recollection of their experiences, but then spoke in cryptic riddles and abstract, spiritual metaphors, indecipherable to me, and, judging from the epidemic of visible confusion in the room, indecipherable to most others.

Though I had cleared the first hurdle of remembering my visions, I worried about the second hurdle of explaining them. Because of the otherworldly and borderline ineffable nature of Ayahuasca visions, explaining them using the limited capacity of language proved unanimously difficult. A perplexing language barrier stood tall between everyone, even between native English speakers, and I noticed that the numerous non-native speakers — already well versed in scaling language barriers and explaining ideas using a limited linguistic toolset — performed significantly better than their native English counterparts.

Despite the linguistic difficulties, and despite our initial bashfulness, a strong bond of camaraderie blossomed as we shared our experiences and thoughts. Trust began to build, and people began to open up, which brewed a steadily intensifying emotional gravity in the room. A safety net of communal empathy alleviated fear and nervousness. Those who managed to recall and articulate their experiences poured out their hearts in amazing displays of candidness, putting their vulnerabilities out in the open, admitting their weaknesses and faults in front of a room full of strangers.

Several people wept uncontrollably as they dragged us with them along the jagged depths of despair, recounting their heartbreaking histories of self-destructive addictions, horrific past traumas, and lifelong battles against crippling psychological strangleholds. But their sorrowful weeping transitioned into tears of joy as they hoisted us back into the heights of relief and inspiration, telling of their unimaginable progress the past two days, the very idea of which they had almost given up on. The range and power of their emotions overwhelmed several listeners, and they too sobbed uncontrollably. The emotions nearly overwhelmed me as well, and I teetered on the brink of crying, surprised to find my throat parched and constricting upon itself, my chest fluttering, and my eyes welling up.

Compounding these emotions, guilt weighed down on me as I listened to the testimonials of my courageous cohorts. I realized that many of them had come to the retreat out of desperation, which dwarfed my reasons of curiosity and introspection. I realized that my seat in the circle could have been filled by someone with a serious need to be there, someone like the brave participant who openly admitted the shambles into which her life had unknowingly collapsed.

"Crazy thinkin' about it, but back home I couldn't even see what my addiction was doin' to me. If I hadn't come to this retreat, I would've been dead within a year...no doubt."

Despite the emotional testimony of my predecessors, and despite the full-grown men and women weeping around me, I somehow managed not to cry when my turn came. My voice quivered as I retold the abridged version of my visions, in terms of experiencing my past actions through the eyes of others and feeling how it affected them. My meager offering paled in comparison to the heart-wrenching contributions of my peers, but as far as presentable material, it was all I had.

The sharing session concluded in stark contrast to how it began, and we all embraced in a prolonged group hug that infused in me an unshakable abundance of positivity and optimism, the likes of which I couldn't find in recent memory. On the walk back to my hut, I shivered from repeated pulses of delight that tickled me from head to toe, and I felt weightless upon the jungle paths. My state of bliss lingered throughout the day and into the evening when we gathered again in the dining area, the morning's musty odor of collective apprehension now replaced with a refreshing air of unity and communal bonding.

We closed the night with lively heart-to-heart conversations while savoring a delectable candlelit meal, our first dinner in two days, and our last dinner for the next three.

Third Night with Ayahuasca

As I sat at the breakfast table munching on eggs and gruel and fresh fruit, the woman sitting across from me squirmed in her seat, restless and uncomfortable from the dozens of fresh glowing red welts that speckled her skin. Hordes of mosquitoes had feasted on her during the night, while an ungodly gang of other insects had also mercilessly bit or stung her, seemingly just for the sport of it.

From the breakfast table sidelines, a gentleman of questionable tact pointed out her condition's resemblance to chickenpox. She barked a gruff assertion that she did not have chickenpox, and I silently concurred, noting the wild variance in welt size, some as large as the hardboiled egg yolks that I shoveled into my mouth.

She twisted her face into a scowl, torn between her better judgment and the unbearable urge to scratch, and she fidgeted in self-restraint, itchy and miserable, grumbling about the ineffectiveness of DEET-free insect repellent. Her misfortune served as a reminder to stay diligent in my defenses, and that here in the jungle, nature had home field advantage. I offered my condolences, and the staff advised that the shamans could concoct a plant-based jungle remedy to help soothe her itching. She rushed to clear her plate and darted off to the shamans' walk-in pharmacy, which, only three days prior, had served as the makeshift altar for our self-induced vomiting.

After breakfast I nursed a cup of tea while pondering the evening's upcoming ceremony and whether to increase my dosage. The medium-sized dose from the second ceremony, though extreme, still felt within my limits, and a cautious confidence encouraged me to challenge myself.

Across the room sat two staff members, a man and a woman, both well experienced with the brew. Their combined wisdom piqued my curiosity, so I cleared my dishes and made a brief stop at their table.

"A question, if I may?"

They both looked up and waited in silence for me to continue.

"Of all your experiences with Ayahuasca, was there ever a ceremony where you felt like you drank too much?"

Neither responded immediately, instead turning to one another, both yielding to the other. He motioned "ladies first" with a nod of the head and a chivalrous open palm in her direction. After prolonged consideration, she rambled off an enthusiastic and detailed but drawn-out and meandering soliloquy as she waxed nostalgic about specific ceremonies and the experiences therein. In sharp contrast, he quipped a terse one-word response, which reinforced the conclusion of her roundabout answer.

"No."

His unblinking eyes and rigid confidence solidified my decision.

"All right, then tonight I guess I'm going for the large cup!"

I thanked them for their counsel and then bid farewell with a smile.

Images of chickenpox welts danced in my mind as I spent the remainder of the day in the refuge of my mosquito net, mentally preparing myself for the repulsive chore of choking down a large dose, and preparing myself for the ensuing epic journey. I set aside my extreme aversion to vomiting and gave myself permission to puke if necessary, noting that several participants claimed that vomiting itself felt therapeutic. Most importantly, I reminded myself that after strapping in for the ride, there would be no getting off until the end, and that no matter what visions may come, my only good option would be acceptance.

Night fell, and anxious excitement tickled me as I sat on my mat awaiting my turn. The staff summoned me to the center of the hut, and I choked down a hideous four gulps of the brew, pausing liberally between gulps. Nausea hit instantly, but surprisingly comparable to that of the medium dose. The other participants received their doses, and then almost immediately after the staff extinguished the lanterns, the Ayahuasca hit me with surprising force.

Empty blackness expanded infinitely in all directions as I stood with my hands by my sides and my emotional state as calm as the void that surrounded me. I glimpsed down to find myself wearing an unfamiliar black suit — a perfect fit, not a crease to be found, tailor-made from exquisite fabrics, luxurious beyond anything I had ever worn. A masterful four-in-hand knot topped off the matching tie which draped from my neck like a frozen waterfall of black silk, running toward my matching shoes of paradoxical comfort and formal elegance.

Upon an invisible altar a short distance in front of me, an open casket levitated at eye level with its occupant just out of sight from my low vantage point. The casket's lacquered mahogany, sleek and polished, glimmered under an unidentifiable light source that illuminated both the casket and me without casting any shadows. Meticulous embroidery and folds of satin cloth billowed out from the casket's open half, adorning the inside with holy white cushioning that decoratively spilled out and cascaded down the outside.

A requiem of profound silence muted the rustling of my suit pants and the clacking of my dress shoes as I ascended the invisible steps of the altar. Nothing about the desolate vigil offered any clues toward the identity of the departed, and none of my friends or family back home suffered ill health, but in the same way that one can read bad news from a person's eyes before any words are spoken, I intuitively knew whose cold body lay before me, even before the pale, lifeless face of my father came into view.

He wore a subtle smile — not the crafty work of an embalmer who wrangled it out of rigor mortis, but a genuine smile — slightly mischievous, captured like a photograph taken at just the right moment. His closed eyelids sealed in the final sense of serenity that had aided him in discarding his physical body. Fingers interlocked, his folded hands across his chest symbolized his absolute content: that he hadn't struggled or resisted, but rather, with graceful acceptance, had acknowledged that his time had come.

I rested my hands upon the casket's pillowed lining, and I yearned to latch on, to forestall his departure. But as I gazed down upon his expired body, its exuding tranquility penetrated through my eyes and through my chest, encouraging me to let go, and empowering me with the same peaceful acceptance that he had exercised in his departure.

The vision forced me to confront the strange and unfamiliar concept of losing a loved one, and I realized for the first time in my life that I had subconsciously built a wall of stone around myself as an emotional defense mechanism. The impenetrably thick and insurmountably tall barrier protected me from the pain of losing loved ones, but at the cost of isolating myself from the very loved ones whom I feared losing. I recognized that this defense mechanism derived from my fear of intimacy — my fear of vulnerability — and I realized that ever since the passing of my grandparents, I had been subconsciously distancing myself from my father, and from the pain of losing him, because even though he likely still had many more years ahead of him, he was also likely the next in line.

In the same way that the moment of lucidity naturally triggers the collapse of a dream, my mere recognition of the emotional stone wall triggered its self-destruction. I closed my eyes and saw a spider web of thin cracks ripping through the barrier that surrounded me. The stone and mortar popped and wedged itself apart under its own weight. Chunks of stone tumbled down like sheets of melting polar ice caps, and beaming sunbursts of orange and yellow light poured in through the crumbling wall's fissures, dousing me in a warm, euphoric shower of liberation. My knees buckled under the weight of emotional overload, and I felt like I had stepped outside into the springtime sunshine after a lifetime of dark and wintry solitary confinement.

I drew in a long, deep breath through my nostrils, exhaled slowly through my mouth, opened my eyes, and once again gazed upon my father's discarded body. My subconscious whispered to me the inevitable words that I didn't want to hear, but which I knew to be true:

"Time to say goodbye."

Both he and I had always preferred to keep our conversations concise, so rather than a long and drawn-out farewell, I simply leaned over and planted a short kiss on his bald head. His cold and rubbery flesh left a salty taste on my lips, triggering a flashback of us watching The Simpsons *together, and a quote from Homer:*

"It's like kissing a peanut!"

The phrase transported me into the depths of long-forgotten childhood memories, and I found my little-boy self sitting next to my father on our living room couch. The television's glow illuminated our faces as we exploded into laughter together, exchanging squinted glances of mutual delight. Upon my lap sat the remains of our ritual Sunday night bag of microwave popcorn, and the flickering television

86

reflected off the buttery oil that coated my fingers as I licked them one by one.

But the memory quickly collapsed, and I found myself back beside my father's casket. The sound of our laughing echoed in layers, fading away into the dark surroundings of endless emptiness, and so too faded away my instinct to latch on. I smiled and withdrew my hands from the casket, straightened my back, gazed down upon him one last time, and allowed myself to finally admit the inevitable regarding my father back home.

"He is going to die one day."

Acceptance and peace of mind flooded my entire being, exterminating every trace of the resistance and denial that had consumed me. A cool tingling of serenity fluttered in my chest and diffused throughout my torso, alleviating a tremendous, malignant pressure that had poisoned my body unbeknownst to me. My next breath startled me with the intensity of its rejuvenation, as if I were taking in my first breath of life. An irrepressible smile of peacefulness widened across my face, while my father's discarded body, still wearing the same mischievous grin, permanently smiled back.

I bid him a silent and loving farewell, which triggered the accelerated rotting of his corpse like time-lapse nature footage of a decomposing carcass. His well-pressed suit and tie disintegrated, and the pale, wrinkled flesh of his naked torso faded to dark shades of moldy green and bruised purple. Globs of flesh drooped and slid off his face like melting rubber, exposing his withered jaw muscles and his lifeless eyes which stared into the empty skies above. From beneath the surface of his rotting skin, a writhing frenzy of worms and maggots erupted outward, eating their way to the surface from the inside, spilling out in a wriggling avalanche of coagulated blood and yellow pus. Within seconds the insatiable swarm devoured every piece of his *soft tissue, and then immediately vanished, leaving only his frail skeleton. His rib cage collapsed on itself, setting off a chain reaction of brittle crumbling as his skeleton disintegrated into dust and accumulated into an elongated pile upon the casket's soiled interior. With no urn for his ashes and no pallbearers for his casket, my father's remains simply faded away into darkness, and I stood alone in the infinite black void.*

My point of view rose out of my body like a free-floating video camera and swung around to look myself in the face. My physical body stared with curious eyes as I stared back with equal curiosity, and neither of us made a move or a sound. Though lobotomized of its consciousness and bereft of its capacity for communication, my physical body still glimmered with the sentience and intellect of a higher primate.

From intimately close I watched my physical body age in fast forward, years per second. Healthy, vibrant skin tones drained from my flesh and faded to an irregular patchwork of pale and sickly blotches, while unsightly liver spots erupted upon my face and neck. My rapidly weathering flesh sagged, and my cheeks drooped to reveal bloodshot pits of exhaustion below my eyes. My abundant head of hair thinned out to baldness, each strand wilting as it faded from brown to gray to white and then fell like drought-stricken crops from the arid terrain of my wrinkled scalp. My eyebrows thickened into a tangled mess of steel wool, and wiry strands of silver hair sprouted like unruly weeds from my nostrils and ear canals. My yellow, sunken eyes shriveled up like dried oysters, barely clinging to life as they retreated into their wrinkled caverns.

For a fraction of a second, short enough to make me question if I truly saw it, my father's face flashed before me on the head of my withering self.

My perspective zoomed out for a wider view as the rapid decay continued eating away at my body, wearing it down to that of a decrepit old man, indistinguishable from a fresh corpse. Polluted with dark, asymmetrical moles and stained with continents of ghastly liver spots, my flesh drooped like a withered balloon haphazardly strewn over my fragile skeleton. My hunched torso wobbled side to side, and my legs buckled under the miniscule weight of my emaciated body riddled with atrophy. Heavy breathing escalated to labored breathing. Labored breathing escalated to wheezing. Wheezing escalated to gasping. Gasping petered out into intermittent respiratory spasms.

My cadaverous body whimpered its final breath and then froze in place as its eyelids convulsed shut like rickety theater curtains stuttering to a close on the final scene of my life. Instant rigor mortis seized my slouching corpse and froze my gangly arms in place against my protruding hip bones. As if strapped to an invisible gurney steered by an invisible mortician, the gaunt remains of my body reclined back into a horizontal resting position befitting of a corpse. The pointy vertebrae of my parabolic spine jutted out and nearly tore through the raggedy flesh of my back, and my hunching neck and shoulders refused to relax, permanently frozen stiff in a half sit-up.

From the surrounding blackness, my father's wooden casket materialized and enclosed my corpse, just as it had enclosed his, upon an invisible altar. My consciousness floated in for a closer view of my expired body, and I gazed down upon it just as I had upon my father's, while my corpse succumbed to the same fate and rotted away in fast forward. I watched in peaceful silence as a slimy mass of writhing grubs burrowed out from beneath my decomposing flesh, devoured the putrid, discolored tissue, picked my bones clean, and left only brittle fossils of my skeletal remains, which then crumbled to dust. The soiled casket faded away, taking with it the small pile of my powdered remains, leaving my consciousness all alone and buoyant in the eternal sea of dark silence.

From the abyss of my subconscious, a microscopic bubble of thought ascended toward my conscious mind, tickling me like a tiny belch trickling up my esophagus. The tiny thought bubble reached the surface of my consciousness and then burst with a short pop, spilling its soft, audible contents into the silence of the surrounding void:

"I am also going to die one day."

The words echoed into infinity as their raw truth resonated in relentless surround sound, all-encompassing and inescapable, forcing me to confront my own mortality. I chuckled at the absurdity and futility of denial, and then with wholehearted sincerity I acknowledged the inevitable, repeating the words back to myself.

"Yep. I'm going to die one day. That's just the way it goes."

As with the acknowledgment of my father's mortality, the affirmation of my own mortality triggered an explosion of rapturous relief that gushed outward from within me, like the unstoppable waters of an exploded dam. The raging flood spilled out of me in all directions, engulfed me, and then poured back into me in cyclical waves, each one taking my breath away.

The hyper-realistic vision converged with the physical world, and my physical body gasped and writhed in ecstasy. I teetered on the verge of moaning, deterred only by the silence of the room. The shamans still sat in silence in the center, meaning that the ceremony had only just begun, and that despite my already severe intoxication, the peak was yet to come.

A new vision soon unfolded before my closed eyes, even more lucid than the last.

An organic, breathing background of soothing pastels swirled around me as I sat naked in lotus position. Amorphous colored patches bled into each other and transitioned from one pleasant hue to another. I spun my head around to discern if perhaps I sat inside a towering lava lamp, but my own train of thought sounded foreign and impersonal. Confusion threatened to creep in, so I cleared my mind and focused my attention on experiencing the vision, rather than analyzing it.

My quiet mind and quiet surroundings lacked anything sexually provocative, and despite my complete absence of psychological arousal, I felt my member growing heavy, inflating with blood, extending in length and expanding in girth as it stood erect. Though physically attached to me, it felt like a separate entity wielding its own will and sentience, like a conjoined twin beyond my control. It quickly doubled and then tripled in length, swelling to unreal girth as it slithered all the way up my abdomen like a curious python.

It reached chest height, engorged thicker than my forearm, and the Cyclops serpent ogled my lips in silent lust as I gripped the base with both hands in a futile attempt to restrain the beast. It purred with a low humming that vibrated throughout my torso, and the shaft pulsated with formidable strength as it climbed further, expanding wider than my grip and forcing my fingers apart. I watched in disbelief as it climbed to eye level and swelled to comical proportions, engorged larger than the head upon my shoulders. It bulged with lustful anticipation and teemed with an inexorable craving for warm, moist friction.

Although tempted to steer away the vision in favor of something more introspective, I knew that the Ayahuasca had control of me, not the other way around. I also knew that attempting to flee the vision would likely backfire and end with my own preposterous erection orally raping me. So instead of resisting, I accepted the vision but pointed out the obvious impracticality of fellatio:

"There is no way that thing is going to fit inside me."

From the skies of swirling colors above, four glimmering dragonflies descended in perfect parallel lines to meet me at eye level. They paused in silent salutation, and their shining iridescent colors swirled about them like liquid fireworks, in gorgeous contrast against the lava lamp background of fluid rainbows. They entranced me with their dazzling vibrancy and grace, diverting my attention away from the throbbing monster that sprouted from between my legs.

The four dragonflies drifted toward me with the flawless unison of synchronized swimmers, and they gently clasped the four corners of my mouth. My jawbone unhooked itself from my skull, with the same audible pop and gratifying sensation of a healthy chiropractic neck crack. The dragonflies stretched my elastic lips and mouth apart to impossible lengths, twice the width of my skull, and then slid the warm blanket of my flesh taut over the head of my massive python erection, securing my lips into a vacuous grip around the entire watermelon-sized bulb. Its enormous surface area ignited with tenfold the sensation of fellatio in the physical world, and an irrepressible moan erupted from my lungs but instantly died in my throat, stifled by my bulging mouthful of myself. The incredible sensation obliterated my higher consciousness, and carnal instincts took rigid possession of me.

The dragonflies released their hold on my lips and retreated a short distance to scrutinize their work. Satisfied, they ascended in silence back into the twirling sea of colors above, and as they disappeared out of sight, a faint drizzle fell from the rainbow skies. The droplets coalesced in slow motion — thicker than rainwater, with the warmth of body heat — dribbling like saliva down my face, down my shoulders, and down my arms. The clear, iridescent precipitation reflected the whirlpool of background rainbow colors as it accumulated upon my skin and coated me with the scent and sleekness of female arousal.

I wrapped both arms into a bear hug around the trunk of my erection, pulling it tight against my chest and embracing it like a passionate lover. Its warmth melded with that of my bare torso as I slid my clutching arms up and down the monstrous shaft, slathering it with the liquid silk that now poured down and crashed upon my naked body. The profuse lubrication ignited raging sexual exhilaration that forced an involuntary quiver with every bear-hug stroke.

Without warning, an ocean of blinding light flooded my vision, and I felt my consciousness peeling apart from my physical body like Velcro. The rampant sexual energy and intense gratification still coursed through me, unwavering even as my consciousness detached from the tactile receptors of my body. My weightless and formless consciousness levitated in a blinding white limbo of sexual ecstasy for a brief moment before the oppressive brightness subsided and revealed an entirely new setting.

My blurred vision came into focus deep inside a vast sultry cavern, surrounded by vibrant rosy pink. Blanketing warmth colluded with a steamy air of sexual intimacy to further intoxicate me with maddening arousal. Like liquefied jewels, drops of sparkling moisture seeped from the soft pink walls, precipitating into a thick humidity of carnal lust. From the dark reaches of the cavern's unseen entrance, the bulging head of an unyielding erection pried open the elastic walls of the cavern and barreled down on me. The pink tunnel hugged the glistening shaft, which I recognized as my own, now cured of its elephantiasis.

From my detached, microscopic vantage point, the firm shaft dwarfed me like a blimp as it plunged into the canal of snug warmth. The bulging head's millions of hypersensitive nerve endings each pulsated with a unique pixel of brilliant golden-yellow, each one feeding a stream of orgasmic pleasure into my consciousness. The wild and tangible sensation of flesh gliding against flesh rivaled the realism of intercourse in the physical world, and the moist friction of every inward thrust and every outward withdrawal ignited a mesmerizing sea of glowing pixels upon the shaft. Harder thrusting amplified the staggering sensations and intensified the exploding firework illuminations as the shaft rammed in and out like an enormous piece of organic machinery.

A rude grumbling bellowed through my innards and snapped me back into the physical world, where I discovered to my dismay that I was pitching a tent. Embarrassment overwhelmed me as I covered the bulge with my folded hands, but my embarrassment turned to relief when I realized that the night already cloaked me in darkness and hid from view the inappropriate spectacle between my legs.

Sharp and painful intestinal cramping assisted me in swiftly deflating my erection and dismantling the tent. More gurgling bellowed from within me, fully audible over the singing shamans, their state of progress unknown to me. My self-inflicted large dose of Ayahuasca wrenched my guts, and I writhed on my mat in hopes that squirming would help the wretched pangs pass through me, but to no avail. Physical discomfort overrode my intoxication, and for several long, uncomfortable minutes, complete sobriety dominated me.

My nausea snickered at me as it crept to new heights, surpassing the moderate levels of previous ceremonies. I sat up and pawed in the dark until my right knuckles bumped against the thick plastic of my vomit pail. As a precaution, I placed the pail on my lap, but immediately an avalanche of fatigue buried my nausea and vaporized my sobriety. I cast my vomit pail back off to the side as I reclined onto my back and once again entered the world of visions.

A disjointed, rambling train of thought polluted my mind with nonsensical mutterings that emulated my own voice but originated from somewhere unknown, distant and foreign. Jumbled words intersected each other and slurred together, half incomprehensible, racing faster than I could follow.

Accompanying the incoherent babbling, a confusing montage of unrelated, transparent imagery flashed around me like a surrounding wall of holographic monitors. Some monitors faced me head on, while others faced me slanted diagonally, some oriented right side up, others upside down, all of them brimming with urgency and demanding my attention. I looked toward the monitor straight ahead, and it slurped me up into an immersive maze of foreign city streets that overwhelmed me with the dread of being late and lost. The monitor then spit me out, and an adjacent one slurped me up into its own immersive world where an unmanned circus of wild predators growled and snarled at me. That monitor likewise spit me out, and another one slurped me up into its upside-down world where a dizzying merry-go-round of impatient faces twirled around and leered at me with disgruntled, unblinking eyes awaiting responses to questions unknown. That monitor spit me out, and another one slurped me up into its world where an enormous factory of malfunctioning machinery wailed with critical alarms that demanded remediation, but the unfamiliar components and gadgets confounded me.

Once again spit back out into center stage, I stood surrounded by the wall of confusing monitors that all screamed for my attention. The nonsensical and now deafening foreign stream of consciousness still rambled in my mind and bombarded me as I tried to focus on one monitor at a time, but none of them made sense.

A second foreign stream of consciousness activated, layering on top of the first and rambling with its own incoherent soliloquy. The two shouted louder and louder, fighting with each other and tugging my attention in opposite directions. As the unintelligible shouting tag-teamed me in surround sound, a second wall of holographic monitors appeared and flashed on top of the first. Like the dueling streams of consciousness, both layers of monitors demanded my attention, but whether I gave it to the first or to the second, confusion and information overload disoriented me.

My native stream of consciousness butted in and spewed forth its own disjointed, loud-mouthed, rambling mess of verbal diarrhea.

"Would I be able to restart my old career if I had to? Do I still have control of my bowels? Was it a bad idea to spend all this money to come to Peru? Whose thoughts are these? Should I even bother pursuing intimate relationships? What the hell is this brew doing to me? Did that damn floral bath give me typhoid? Who the hell are these shamans? What if I soil myself? Have I lost my sanity?"

Each worrisome utterance resonated in the echo chamber of my mind and accumulated into a vibrating, towering stack of layered worry upon worry. I instinctively latched on to each thought, desperate to resolve them all, and one by one their toxicity seeped into me, poisoning me with fear. At the same time, the dueling streams of consciousness pestered me with their incessant tempest of babbling, and the nonstop visual intrusion of holographic distractions blared at me for attention. The pandemonium culminated into a migraine of visible noise like the snowy chaos of an old television without a signal, and I squirmed in a desperate attempt to ward off the unbearable mental assault.

Barely audible over the ensuing mental anarchy, in my own voice, three soft syllables fell upon my ears, landing with a feather's touch.

"Surrender."

I repeated the word back to myself, likewise in a whisper. The nearly inaudible utterance detonated a nuclear explosion of clarity in my mind, launching a seismic wave of silence that demolished the rampant mental noise and neutralized its toxicity. The layered holographic monitors shattered like mirrors in zero gravity and propelled tiny, glistening shards of thought outward in every direction, off into infinity, leaving in their wake a background of heavenly white. The radiating light surrounded me from every angle, and its invigorating warmth, like sunshine upon my skin, instantly filled me with bliss. I floated weightless and ecstatic in the silent ocean of light with no sense of orientation or direction. The concepts of right side up, upside down, and sideways all ceased to exist, and every direction seemed to be right side up.

A few rust-colored blotches, resembling spray paint on a wall, tainted the otherwise immaculate white that encompassed me. I intuitively recognized that the blotches represented negative thoughts — worries and fears, regrets and anxiety — to which I still clung, and that my subconscious latching on to them had tainted the natural state of my mind. Like a flamboyant magician with a cape and magic wand, I twirled about and vaporized the blotches one by one with a silent abracadabra and exaggerated flick of my wrist, and each blotch exploded into a small plume of beige dust that disintegrated into glimmering nothingness.

The freshly sanitized patches poured forth with illumination and bombarded me with intense rays of bliss that took my breath away. I gasped a massive inhale that drew in life-giving oxygen along with a bewildering cornucopia of positivity, both emotional and physical — the heartwarming joy of friendship and love, the tranquilizing serenity of a skillful massage, the electrifying pride of a hard-fought accomplishment, the exhilarating refreshment of a cool breeze on a hot summer day — all contained within a simple breath.

The extraordinary rush of positivity coursed through my entire being, permeating every nook and cranny in my mind and body. The thrill of a simple inhale astonished me, and I gasped a second time before exhaling the first, instantly belching out the second gasp like a tiny hiccup, which tickled me with jubilation. My limbs trembled, and I shook them to collect myself before slowly expelling the massive breath, casting out every trace of residual negativity, banishing it from my body.

My point of view zoomed out from the side of my cranium and swirled around to an out-of-body perspective a few paces away, where I watched myself eradicate the last remaining blotch, and in that same moment, my body imploded into a cloud of thin, sparkling white smoke. Brilliant rays of light poured out from behind the plume's opaque silhouette and arrested my attention. Like the morning sun beaming from behind a horizon of clouds, a glowing white orb rose from the dissipating smoke. Wide and oval, solid and dense, heavy like marble and small enough to fit in the palms of my hands, the levitating orb emanated an unimaginable purity that humbled me with its flawless brilliance. Humility and awe combined with my already teeming ecstasy, and the emotional alchemy exploded into a euphoric state of such unbearable, suffocating intensity that I assumed I must have died upon my mat in the jungle. I felt no trace of the physical world, my physical body, my memories, my sense of time, or my sense of self — only the infinite lightness of unadulterated awareness, absolute freedom, and complete detachment from everything.

The brilliant orb appeared inanimate and yet seemed to stare at me with profound intelligence. From somewhere distant and unknown, a question echoed into my awareness, in my own voice.

"What is this orb?"

In the same instant that I perceived the question, a clairvoyant response likewise echoed in my own voice.

"Pure consciousness."

The confident response spawned a sudden genesis of revelatory knowledge in my mind — new, raw information that somehow downloaded itself directly into my consciousness, bypassing the usual interfaces of language and sensory input. A strange confidence inside me asserted that my consciousness was not just an individual entity, but rather part of a collective consciousness that connects every living thing. I suddenly recognized that through the discarding of my physical body, the dismantling of my ego, and the detachment from all thought, I now existed in a formless state of pure consciousness, and that I could freely traverse the collective consciousness to tap into the personal perspective of anyone, anywhere. Though utterly new to me, the revelations somehow struck me as ancient common knowledge as timeless as the universe itself.

The bliss of total detachment persisted as my consciousness soared at warp speed to the boundaries of outer space and then slammed to an abrupt stop at the apex of the universe, where I gazed down upon a vast ocean of twinkling galaxies and solar systems. I pondered the countless possibilities of whose consciousness to connect with, and then the smirking face of an estranged friend flashed before me, so I set course for his consciousness.

A hailstorm of stars tore past me in a flurry of streaking lights as I travelled at hyper-speed through the universe. The blinding light of whizzing stars culminated in a sheet of solid white, then transitioned into the light of fluorescent bulbs: long thin tubes suspended in the ceiling above an office cubicle in which I sat. On the desk in front of me, two mountains of cluttered papers teetered on the brink of avalanche, sandwiching a computer monitor smeared with fingerprints, the plastic perimeter of its frame littered with faded and peeling sticky notes of illegibly scrawled passwords. An ambient murmur of chatter overlaid the persistent clickety-clack of fingertips tapping keyboards, occasionally complemented by the hum of a printer warming up and spewing out a stack of pages. The smells of Freon, coffee, hand sanitizer, and excessive cologne and perfume wafted through the recycled office air.

As a spectator tapped into the consciousness of my estranged friend, I watched from his perspective while he covertly browsed online for sports bloopers, amusing animal tricks, and anything else that offered a distraction from the drudgery of life in his cubicle. He repeatedly looked over his shoulder, always on high alert, trying to dodge his bosses while also trying to dodge doing any real work, and at the sound of approaching footsteps he hid away his online diversions with a swift and stealthy click of the mouse. He hadn't changed a bit since the last time we met, and his sneaky shenanigans delighted me to no end.

Intense cramping pain jolted me from the vision, and I locked my back into a spastic arch while enduring what felt like an agitated pufferfish scraping through my intestines. Stifled grunts and labored exhales punctuated my repeated assertions to myself that everything passes, and I wrestled my sour face into a smile, unwilling to let the pain detract from my newfound euphoria. My self-assurances soon proved correct, and the abdominal cramping fizzled out with a gaseous whimper. I widened my smile, relaxed my back, and then plummeted back into the world of visions.

Blurry, indistinguishable shapes and colors undulated as if viewed through rippling waves of crystal-clear water. Lush green patches bordered long stretches of sandy-beige and vibrant cerulean blue. Flesh-colored dots speckled the scene, strewn about like flecks of paint thrown onto canvas with erratic flicks of the brush. The perplexing vision arrested my attention as it slowly faded into focus, but I struggled to make sense of it.

"What, are those dots supposed to be people? On the beach? Where am I? What is the meaning of this..."

My instinctual desire to understand the blurry scene took hold of me, and I continually drifted further and further away from my blissful state of total detachment. The harder I tried to understand the vision, the more it confused me, and the invigorating warmth of euphoria faded away into an irritating itch of frustration.

At the same time, a distant and unrelated throng of marauding mental noise encroached on my fading peace of mind. I tensed up and resisted the commotion as it barreled down on me, but a series of incoherent conversations in my own voice penetrated my consciousness. My pristine mental state of serenity from only moments ago deteriorated into shambles, now cluttered by worthless mental garbage, onto which I clung like an impoverished hoarder. I grimaced and groaned in search of an escape, but then I remembered the key to my mental salvation, and I whispered it to myself with a smile.

"Surrender. Let it all go."

The mere utterance ignited a deafening explosion of angelic soprano and falsetto — a resounding choir that obliterated all mental noise — and the blinding white light of euphoria flooded back in, bleaching the dirtied walls of my mind.

My heart rate soared, and I trembled from electrifying pulses of relief that surged through me in waves. Opening my eyes pulled me back into the physical world, where I silently gasped for air and then realized that I had been holding my breath. Pitch black darkness filled my jittery vision, and dead silence filled the room. Time had left me behind, marching on for several hours without me. The shamans had finished singing, the ceremony had ended, and severe intoxication still dominated me.

Fatigue restrained me to my mat, and I spent what felt like an hour floating on clouds of bliss, muttering "surrender" to myself. Each utterance triggered two simultaneous surges, one of supreme mental euphoria that annihilated every trace of negativity from my mind, and one of paralyzing physical euphoria that originated in my chest, then pulsated outward to each limb, passionately masturbating every cell in my body. Each simple utterance took my breath away, and each gasping inhale amplified the already enormous sensations that then skyrocketed off the charts.

The throes of ecstasy immobilized me, and I planned to spend the night in the ceremonial hut, but soon sobriety and a vague sense of time trickled back into my consciousness. The discomfort of my flattened mat eclipsed my waning euphoria, while my congested bowels begged for evacuation, forcing me to change plans and start the arduous journey to my hut. But this time I started the journey with some confidence, because I had played the game before, and I knew the winning strategy: balance, baby steps, patience, and focus.

I gathered my bedding supplies, shuffled to the exit and down the steps, secured my shoes on my feet, and then set out on the dark jungle path, in a record-breaking five minutes, without even a wobble. The perilous pitfalls no longer posed a threat now that I had memorized where to step, and I progressed through the uneven terrain with a cautious yet confident snail's pace, free from the anxiety of previous nights.

As I approached the porcupine tree — the jungle marker that signaled the approaching finish line of my hut — a sudden, instinctive alarm of imminent danger stopped me in my tracks. My sense of hearing, still heightened by Ayahuasca, picked up on rhythmic, highly concentrated, powerful gusts of air — stealthy and nearly inaudible over the jungle symphony — originating from directly in front of me, only a few paces away. Before I could elevate my gaze from the dirt path, my peripheral vision glimpsed a blur of flapping wings soaring at me through the air, cloaked by the darkness of the jungle.

Adrenaline and the residual effects of Ayahuasca blended into a confusing cocktail of clumsy hyper-alertness as time crashed to a screeching halt. My instinct to duck and cover conflicted with the real threat of losing my balance, toppling over, falling into the porcupine tree and mangling myself upon its spines, dying for a second time in the same gruesome fashion. I froze in place, lowering my head the few centimeters that I could, while hunching my shoulders in desperate hope that the unknown bird of prey would spare my scalp.

The massive blur of winged darkness swooped just above my head, and I clenched my sphincter to prevent soiling myself. Terror trembled through me, and I stood in wobbly silence as a tremendous overhead whoosh of air shook the surrounding vegetation into a fluttering frenzy, nearly throwing me off balance. The nearby jungle creatures, perhaps also clenching their sphincters, dared not sing their symphony as the vegetation came to a rest and eerie silence faded in. Several long seconds passed before I allowed myself to exhale, at which point my intoxicated mind insisted that I had just survived a pterodactyl attack.

I lumbered back to my hut, then headed straight to the bathroom for what I hoped to be a quick pit stop. Despite the evening's painful, sloshy warning signs both audible and physical, my bowel movement glided out firm and healthy, plopping into the sawdust below with a graceful thump. I waited for several minutes, thinking that the maelstrom of diarrhea lay in ambush, poised to strike at any moment, but it never came — only wretched plumes of nauseating gas.

Back at my bed, I slid under the draped mosquito netting and then crashed into an awkward position lying face down, head not on any of my three pillows, arms and legs sprawled out, waist twisted to the left, neck twisted to the right. My body shut down from exhaustion, but my intoxicated mind continued to churn.

My naked body floated in front of me with its eyes closed, and like a medical diagram, its transparent flesh revealed the internal organs, muscles, skeletal structure, and cardiovascular system. With the scrutinizing eye of a medical examiner, I scoured the inner workings of my physical body, scanning for maladies, and I spotted an abnormal patch of thick, dirty-yellow calcification — a hive of what looked like malignant barnacles crusted on my left shoulder and neck, corresponding to the location of painful and recurring injuries that have plagued me for years.

As I focused my attention on the hive, it glowed with a warm amber aura, as if illuminated by the candlelight of my awareness. Suddenly a sharp and forceful pop rang out, and my transparent body detached itself from the malignant hive, which floated upward as one solid mass. Soft white currents of warm electricity cycled through my neck and shoulder, penetrating through one side and out the other, mending the damaged tissue as the detached hive floated further upward. It paused briefly, levitating above my self-repairing body, and then without warning, the malignant hive exploded like a firecracker, bursting into dust that dissipated into nothingness.

Though visually impressive, the vision felt unconvincing. Awkward silence dominated the room, like when a punchline fails to deliver, and my initial reaction reeked of doubt.

"Poof? That's it? Just like that, I'm healed?"

Though I yearned for it to be true, only time would tell, and I couldn't shake the nagging skepticism that tainted my follow-up comment.

"Hope so..."

Fourth Night with Ayahuasca

"Was there ever a ceremony where you felt like you drank too much?"

"No...(no)...(no)...(no)...(no)..."

The echo of his confident response from the day prior ricocheted back and forth inside my skull as I awoke to a strong feeling that I had drank too much.

I pried open my reluctant eyelids, and in rushed a flood of blurry brightness that forced me to squint. The weak, rickety stilts of my arms trembled as they propped up my torso, and my innards groaned with disapproval of their now vertical orientation.

One at a time, my feet crawled off the bed and dragged my legs with them. I sat slouched on the edge of the bed, exhausted, rubbing my eyes in a vain attempt to wipe away the residual daze of intoxication. In the back of my mind, muffled conversations clouded my thoughts and prevented me from determining if I needed to use the toilet. I failed to reach a verdict after several minutes of futile deliberation, so I declared a mistrial and gave up on the idea.

Micro-fits of vertigo bullied my balance as I attempted to rise. My knees buckled and locked as I wobbled in place like a newborn fawn, fresh out of the womb, unfamiliar with my own limbs. I stood there in my underwear, scratching my head and scanning the inside of my hut as if searching for something — perhaps trying to find the clothes that sat at my feet, or perhaps just trying to find my balance.

An intense yawn stretched my face apart and helped me regain some semblance of myself. I reached down to the floor to grab the same clothing that I had discarded seven hours prior, and I began the laborious task of dressing myself. Each piece of clothing presented its own set of challenges, requiring different feats of coordination and balance that pushed the limits of my current capacity. Partial confidence returned after I successfully dressed myself, but a severe daze of lightheadedness persisted.

Waves of dissociation undulated through me, each crest floating my consciousness a full head-length out of my body and then slowly guiding it back down, returning me to my baseline state of wobbly confusion.

I tried and failed to think of ways to alleviate my symptoms, then defaulted to the panacea of "walk it off" and proceeded out the door.

My body shifted to autopilot and navigated itself to the dining hall, where I found myself sitting at a table and eating slow spoonfuls of breakfast, without a clear recollection of how I got there. The other participants, laughing and engaged in coherent conversation, seemed to suffer none of the mental disarray that afflicted me. I struggled to follow along as one participant recounted the details of soiling himself in bed last night and his frantic use of a nearby towel as an emergency makeshift diaper, which he had stuffed with socks for extra absorption.

Throughout the day, the warmth of the sunlight and the serenity of the jungle invigorated me physically but did little to clear my mental fog. It persisted all the way through nightfall when I found myself back in the ceremonial hut without any vivid memories of the day's activities, once again sitting on my mat and awaiting another dose of Ayahuasca.

My large dose from the previous night had failed to enhance any of the desirable effects, and had instead only worsened the undesirables of disorientation and cramping. My medium dose from the second ceremony felt closer to the sweet spot that I sought — strong visions, but with tolerable side effects — and I decided to scale back to the medium cup for the remaining ceremonies.

From the center of the hut, the staff summoned me to approach the shamans and receive my dose. I kept my gaze low as I approached, to prevent tripping over myself or the protruding floorboards, and I noted the ceremonial accessories and comfort items of my neighbors. They employed a wide variety of spiritual goods — scented oils, hand-rolled ceremonial tobacco, assorted crystals, incense, talismans and charms — all of which contrasted sharply with my lone comfort item of spiritually bankrupt insect repellent.

The shaman poured out my dose one thick glug at a time, and I forced it down my throat as quickly as possible, then returned to my mat. Licking the insides of my mouth failed to wipe away the persistent coat of awful aftertaste, but I did so anyway as a distraction to get me through twenty minutes of waiting in silence, until shapes and colors emerged behind my closed eyes, signaling the beginning of my slow-motion blastoff.

A background of cerulean blue faded in, on top of which symmetrical twirls of forest green danced for me like acrobatic smoke. They branched out to form a complex membrane of glowing jungle colors like multiplying bacteria under a microscope. The flexible soft edges of the membrane expanded and contracted like a breathing organism, and thin tips of branching appendages spiraled around themselves.

The organic patterns coagulated into a vibrant field of lush green grass, surrounded by a thick growth of pristine vegetation, untouched by humankind. Lazy white clouds sailed across a smooth ocean of infinite blue, and the sun graced me with its invigorating yellow rays, warming my body to the core.

I beheld the awe-inspiring landscape in silence, with a pure awareness untainted by words. My consciousness felt primitive and inhuman, devoid of thought or even the ability to think, unequipped to comprehend language, and unequipped to experience anything other than the present moment.

Fertile soil and vibrant blades of soft grass cushioned my weight, and I glanced down at my feet to find two small furry paws and legs supporting my front half. I turned to look behind me and found two more paws attached to furry hind legs propping up my back side, upon which a wild, wagging tail flailed back and forth. The simple joy of being alive overwhelmed me, and I raced in circles chasing my own tail while my tongue flapped out of the side of my snout, slathering my face with an abundant slobber of frenzied exuberance.

A sudden itch behind my ear diverted my one-track mind and nullified the previously imperative task of chasing my own tail. This new and exciting stimulus — a simple itch behind my ear — fully arrested my attention. In one fluid motion I plopped down my rear end while leaning my neck backward, and the gentle claws of my hind leg homed in on the tingling itch, pumping away with a quick series of furious but precise scratching that inflamed me with gratification.

A low rumble off in the distance once again diverted my limited attention, freezing my hind leg mid-scratch as I raised my head and perked up my ears. From the horizon, a small stampede of elephants and giraffes trotted toward me, brimming with the electrifying eagerness of longtime friends reuniting after years apart. Despite their enormity, the majestic creatures sped toward me with fluid grace, gliding across the grassy plain. I leapt into the air and flailed with excitement, twisting and spinning at the apex of my jumps, barking an emphatic salutation. They doubled their pace and bobbed their heads in anticipation, enthralled to see a furry creature as tiny as myself.

My attempt to race toward them resulted in only a slow-paced, hopping waddle, unbefitting of a puppy, and I gazed down to find myself now wearing a natural tuxedo of sleek, glossy black and white feathers. Stubby, flightless, vestigial wings pressed against the sides of my pear-shaped body and sandwiched my belly of smooth white feathers. In place of legs, two tiny webbed birdlike feet protruded directly from the bottom of my body and prohibited me from running. Without the cognitive ability to recognize my own spontaneous metamorphosis, I simply carried on as if I had always been a penguin.

Unwavering excitement fueled my vigorous waddling as I danced in place and bobbed my head in anticipation of the approaching stampede.

A sunburst of fiery orange pulled me from the vision as my neighbor struck a match to light his hand-rolled ceremonial cigarette. The flame illuminated the contours of his face with an orange glow as he puffed, and thick smoke billowed from his mouth. He extinguished the match with a flick of his wrist and disappeared back into the darkness, and I pondered the meaning of my brief zoological vision from moments prior. It struck me as a manifestation of my longing for simplicity in life, as I had often envied the lives of dogs and other animals that presumably spend their entire existence in the present moment, free from the complications and daily woes of modern humans who tend to focus on the past and future.

Amid my introspection, a demonic, guttural gurgling tore through the room, shattering the silence like a brick through glass. The abrupt and heinous eruption offered no forewarnings — no preliminary gagging or dry heaving, no sound of blind hands searching for a vomit pail, no excessive spitting of saliva — only sudden, startling cries of desperation, and the dreadful sound of someone's dilated throat giving birth to a massive glob of gastric agony.

I curled under my blanket and closed my eyes to flee the physical world, but the wretched sounds pursued me into the world of visions.

An unfamiliar face appeared before me, only a few paces away, grimacing in the pangs of distress. He clamped his eyelids shut, unable to open them for fear of the horror he would behold, the horror that tortured him with its slow crawl up his throat, from the depths of his bowels. Along the length of his furrowed and sweaty brow, pronounced wrinkles further deepened with his intensifying cringes. His face heaved, mouth agape, as his neck muscles strained and his veins bulged, all synchronized with the foul noises that poured into the ears of my physical body in the ceremonial hut. Despite his strenuous effort, only a bashful procession of dark stomach acid dribbled from his bottom lip, staining it with Ayahuasca's vile brown hue.

After dry heaving to the brink of exhaustion, my struggling neighbor bellowed out the crescendo of his tragic performance — a gurgling swan song of several grueling seconds during which his body strained to expel his entire digestive tract. His cries intensified and elevated in pitch as if a dense glob of mucus were filling his throat from the bottom up. The concave shape of his vomit pail seemed to act as a megaphone, amplifying both his wailing and the sounds of heavy goo crashing into plastic, sloshing around as additional layers piled on top.

His strained face spewed forth a relentless stream of projectile vomit, spraying inhuman amounts of Ayahuasca-infused gastric juices into the air between us, a mere arm's length away from dousing my entire front side. I recoiled in disgust but fought my instinct to flee, reminding myself that I couldn't run away, that I had to accept and embrace the visions, no matter how unpleasant.

A solid stream of his vomit splashed at my feet as I faced him head-on and fixed my gaze upon the endless fountain of filth pouring from his face. The salvation and bliss of surrendering echoed in my mind as I inhaled a deep breath and then expunged it along with my strong aversion to vomiting, and although the repulsive spectacle before me remained unchanged, my perception of it changed. I no longer saw it as a human body purging the putrid contents of its stomach, but rather I saw it as the objective concept of liquid flowing from an opening, no more or less disgusting than water flowing from a faucet.

My neutral objectivity then transformed into sympathy, and I saw him as my fellow human, in agony and in need of help. My sympathy ballooned and compelled me to console him, and without hesitation I peeled my heels off the sticky vomit-covered floor to walk toward him, my every step squishing down a fresh footprint into the chunky mess that carpeted the dark floor.

Tears leaked from the sides of his eyes clamped shut. Lumpy veins nearly burst as they bulged from his forehead and temples and neck. His strenuous and sustained physical exertion cast his face a ghastly shade of purple. The relentless stream of yellow-brown vomit arched from his mouth like a fountain statue, and he remained oblivious as I stepped directly into his line of fire.

I held my eyes open as his acidic regurgitations splashed against my face. From the black skies above, torrential vomit poured down and crashed upon my body, drenching my hair and clothing. Warm chunks of partially digested food clung to my skin, resisting gravity as they tumbled in slow, sticky summersaults down my arms and down the back of my neck.

His endless flow of vomit raged on, splashing in my face as I reached out both arms and cupped my hands around the back of his straining neck. Vomit ricocheted in all directions off my forehead and eyes and cheeks and mouth as I drew his face in closer to mine, but my sympathetic gesture shut off the valve to his fountain of gastric juices and halted the downpour of vomit from above. He closed his gaping mouth and then stood motionless, making no effort to wipe away the thick and stringy goo that dribbled from his lip and down his chin. I likewise made no effort to wipe his dribbling vomit from my own face, allowing it to run down my brow and into my eyes, down my cheeks and over my lips as I planted a platonic kiss of brotherly love on his vomit-covered lips. Small, soggy chunks of Ayahuasca-soaked regurgitations squished between our lips as I silently assured him that he need not distress, and that everything was okay.

The thick coating of sticky vomit evaporated from our hair and from our drenched bodies. With eyes still closed, he flashed a faint smile as he faded away into the darkness of our surroundings.

I opened my eyes and realized that the shamans were already singing, that mild cramping was jabbing at my innards, and that my forehead was tingling. The singing and the cramping were expected, but the tingling confused me. Because it had been nearly a week since my last proper shower, I assumed that my Ayahuasca-induced heightened sense of touch must be detecting the caked-up layers of dirt and sweat and insect repellent that clogged my pores. I then discarded that reasonable hypothesis in favor of the paranoid assumption that mosquitoes must be tap-dancing on my face.

I attempted to scatter the alleged hordes by twirling a limp-wristed and clumsy swat around my face. I then smacked my palm upon my forehead and wiped the length of my face from top to bottom, but the tingling continued, and I assumed that a cloud of mosquitoes must be dive-bombing my face, deftly maneuvering around my futile swatting.

I sought refuge under the cover of my blanket, pulling it over my head and then wiping my face with the blanket's underside. The tingling stopped, but as I lay on my back, sealed in on all sides, the blanket trapped my warm breath against my face, slowly suffocating me with a stifling mask of humidity. Moments later my forehead started tingling again.

Paranoia asserted that the entire insect kingdom had launched an attack upon me, and that they had infiltrated my stronghold. I considered turning over onto my front side and burying my face in my pillow, but the mere thought of pressure upon my abdomen nauseated me. As with the mosquito attack during that fateful camping trip from my youth, my current circumstances afforded me no good options.

Flashbacks haunted me as I writhed in despair, recalling with renewed clarity the infuriating nuisance of faint but constant buzzing in my ears, the sweltering heat inside the temporary refuge of my tiny sleeping bag, and the sweltering heat inside the family minivan with the windows sealed shut. Panic nearly consumed me, but then a whisper from my subconscious reminded me that I already knew the solution to my predicament: surrender. Like the flip of a switch, simply hearing the word in my head triggered a complete mental shift.

The swirling thoughts of despair faded out, and I tossed my blanket aside, conceding that if insects wanted to eat my face, then I would let them eat my face, without a fight.

My naked body levitated in front of me, just an arm's length away on a backdrop of darkness. Hundreds of mosquitoes and roaches and centipedes swarmed me, blanketing my face with their prickly legs, jockeying for position on the prime real estate of my eyeballs, nostrils, and ear canals. The swarm devoured my flesh like piranhas, with tiny but rapid and voracious bites, annihilating the appetizer of my epidermis. My viewpoint zoomed in for a close-up of a centipede's pointed, curved mandibles tearing out chunks of my eye and shoveling the soft white tissue into the frenzied stubby feelers that surrounded its orifice. Most of the swarm continued ravaging my exposed facial muscles while a lucky minority wriggled and gnawed their way through my eye sockets, up my nostrils, and through my inner ears, bound for the honey pot of brain tissue inside my skull.

The insatiable swarm devoured every piece of soft tissue above my neck, leaving only my dry, empty skull. Their sumptuous feast fueled an immediate population explosion, and their numbers multiplied exponentially. As one collective organism, the swarm moved down my neck and shoulders and arms, flowing like a wave down the length of my body. They devoured my flesh and exposed my muscles underneath, devoured my muscles and exposed my organs underneath, and then devoured my organs, leaving nothing but my skeleton. After picking dry every bone down to my toes, the swarm scuttled off in search of their next meal, and my decimated skeleton collapsed upon itself.

The tingling upon my forehead persisted, but it now felt detached, distant, and impotent. The same irksome sensation that moments prior had nearly ravaged my sanity now existed only as an inconsequential footnote on my physical state of being.

A tempest of liquid and gas echoed through the corridors of my intestines and snarled a forewarning of the imminent bombardment barreling down on my rectum. As I adjusted my position and warmed up my clenching muscles to brace for impact, a sudden melee of guerilla diarrhea struck me by surprise. I slammed on the emergency brakes of my sphincter a millisecond too late, and something squeaked through, possibly just gas, possibly something more.

The immediate threat of explosive diarrhea slowly subsided, but I stayed clenched at full strength in foolish hope that I could somehow slurp up the leakage back into me. Ever-worsening fatigue and physical disorientation had already immobilized me, precluding any possibility of standing up, much less stumbling to the restroom and cleaning the suspected mess from my bottom.

Fear crept in as I realized that the intoxication confined me to lying on my mat for the next few hours, and that if an uncontainable diarrhea emergency struck, I would be powerless to prevent disaster. The worst-case scenario played out in my mind: trapped alive in my sarcophagus, writhing in a pool of my festering feces; the foul stench wafting over to my neighbors, ruining their ceremonies; the staff having to clean my mess and carry me out of the hut mid-ceremony; disgracing myself and spending the remainder of the week unable to look anyone in the eye.

Beads of sweat rolled down my face, partially from anxiety and partially from strenuous, nonstop sphincter clenching. But as I sank deeper into paranoia and fear, once again my subconscious whispered to me in a calm voice.

"Surrender."

From above, I looked upon the pitiful sight of myself lying on my mat in the circle of participants. I watched my tensed body squirming and my woeful scowl contorting in agony, but my subconscious remained calm and encouraged me to simply let go of the fear.

"Go ahead. Soil yourself."

The liberating words echoed with an angelic resonance that smoothed my rigid grimace into a soft smile and relaxed my stiffened body into a comfortable position on my back. I mentally committed myself to confronting my fear, and invisible stirrups supported my calves as I bent my knees and drew them back into birthing position, preparing for detonation. Hesitance placed its cold hand upon my shoulder and inquired if there weren't a more civilized way to go about this, suggesting that I at least disrobe and use my vomit pail as a makeshift toilet to minimize the mess. Without even looking back to acknowledge the inquiry, I brushed the hand of hesitance off my shoulder and resolved to make the spectacle an extravagant bonanza.

I loosened my sphincter valve, and the explosive diarrhea's tremendous pressure instantly dilated me to softball size, from which I blasted out a raging stream of chunky yellow and brown liquid with the consistency of watered-down oatmeal. The blast tore a hole through the fabric of my undergarments and pajamas, spraying in all directions like an unmanned fire hose, ricocheting and splattering off my elevated heels. Within seconds the putrid mess accumulated into a marsh of liquid feces that surrounded me as I lay motionless and carefree on my back. The marsh rose to ear level and nearly seeped into the corners of my eyes before the fire hose of filth slowed to a trickle. The last few spurts petered out, punctuated by a grand finale shotgun blast of flatulence.

Neither the horrific stench nor the putrid sounds caught the attention of my neighbors, who continued undisturbed on their own individual journeys. My soggy mat squished beneath my body as I rocked back and forth, splashing my open palms in the mess and smiling like a toddler playing in a summertime pool. Liquid feces matted down my hair and crusted over, caking onto my head a helmet of dried diarrhea, and without a hint of shame or disgust, I proudly wore it like a crown.

I extended my limbs out straight, pressed them against the floor, and then swung my arms and legs open and closed like windshield wipers, creating snow angels in my filth. Maniacal laughter launched my chest into heaving spasms, and the beaming bright whites of my toothy smile contrasted with my dark blanket of bodily waste as I sloshed around like a pig in mud.

The muffled songs of the shamans barely penetrated my consciousness as I covered my mouth to suppress an eruption of giggling. I worried that my laughing had disturbed my neighbors, but faint moonlight offered just enough illumination to confirm that both of them appeared deeply immersed in their own worlds, so I likewise delved back into my own.

I found myself inside the fully illuminated cavern of my small intestine, flushed of all contaminants. The surrounding crimson and pink inner walls glistened like polished ruby while I floated through my digestive tract, as if riding a raft down a lazy river. In the wake of the diarrhea storm, a profound serenity and godlike cleanliness permeated my intestinal walls, and my subconscious whispered to me 「台風一過」 *("taifuu ikka"), the succinct Japanese idiom referring to the cloudless, immaculate blue skies that follow the wrath of a typhoon.*

Intestinal villi swayed like sea anemones in the gentle current that floated me through the corridors. The complexities of the digestive system astounded me, and I marveled at its interconnected role in the grand machinery of a complex organism. The carnivorous food chain sprung into my mind, and concepts that I had always taken for granted now confounded me: the recursion of organisms that eat organisms that eat organisms; the barbarism of teeth ripping apart the flesh of other living creatures; the vampirism of extracting the nutrients of another living creature in order to sustain oneself; the inevitability that even a herbivore's existence is dependent upon the killing of other living things.

Suddenly my intuition sensed a massive and powerful force barreling down behind me from a great distance. My intuition warned that the approaching mass would bulldoze anything in its path, so I immediately stepped aside and clung to the villi of my intestines. An enormous cloudy bubble of thick moldy-green gas raced toward me and then stormed by like an ambulance with gurgle sirens blaring. The emergency fart zoomed its way rectum-bound, rushing down the twisting corridors of my intestines, leaving behind a thin scattered trail of nauseating particles in its path, but the residual pollution soon dissipated, and I resumed my leisurely float all the way through my large intestine.

The float ended at the barren silo of my rectum, where I assumed that the emergency fart had already smashed its way through to the outside world. I sauntered up to the downward-facing inner wall of my sphincter and rapped a soft, backhanded knock-knock-knock on the firm muscular doorway. The exit chute instantly fell open like the seat of a dunk tank, spewing me out onto an invisible water slide that I rode smiling and laughing with both arms in the air as the wind rushed over my face. The end of the invisible waterslide launched me upward into a high-flying parabolic arch, and I tucked myself into a cannonball before splashing into an Olympic-sized pool of clear water. Glistening white porcelain surrounded me like an oval bowl-shaped mountain range, and the floor of the pool curved into a dark cavern that led downward out of sight. I frolicked and splashed about, unconcerned with the sanitary conditions of swimming in a giant toilet, as carefree as the Peruvian children I had earlier seen playing in the filthy banks of the Nanay River.

A terrible ruckus from outside jolted me back into the physical world and temporarily drowned out the songs of the shamans. Something crashed downward in a free fall from the jungle canopy, snapping twigs and ripping leaves from their branches before smashing to the ground with a solid thud. I froze in place like a frightened animal sensing a predator, and I listened for any clues to explain the commotion, but the jungle fell silent.

My mind raced for an explanation, rattling off a hurried series of unfounded speculations: perhaps a large, canopy-dwelling creature had sighed its last breath of old age, expired in its sleep, and then crashed to the ground below; perhaps one of the ancient jungle trees had amputated a wounded limb and discarded it to the jungle floor; perhaps the crashing had come not from above, but from a toilet-bound participant who had lost his way, blacked out, and then tumbled off the uneven dirt path into the jungle shrubbery.

An unrelenting and oppressive need for explanation cracked the whip on my racing mind like a merciless dog sled driver.

"Think! Think!! What the hell could've caused such a loud crash!?"

My heart thumped in my chest, and as I teetered on the brink of panic, a revelation struck me: that I didn't have to explain anything, that I had created an artificial obligation, and that the loud crash in the jungle was inconsequential.

My subconscious concurred and whispered to me a simple piece of advice:

"Let it be."

The Beatles song of the same title faded in, momentarily eclipsing the songs of the shamans and muting the hysteria in my mind. The repeating lyrics of the refrain took my breath away with each repetition. Those three simple words astonished me with their broad applicability to life in general, and their potent ability to diffuse so many of life's troubles: arguments, worries, anger, regrets, confusion, stress, fears, grief, jealousy, disappointment, grudges — all powerless to the simple idea of letting go.

I smiled and hummed along, but the dissonant songs of the shamans faded back in, clashing with The Beatles.

I opened my eyes and attempted to sit up, but my body refused. The slow carousel of shamans continually passed me by, their precise locations undeterminable by my distorted sense of hearing, their voices sneaking about like singing ninjas in the dark. Trying to interact with the shamans felt futile, so I gave up on that and instead focused my attention inward.

Only faint, scattered swirls of light and color pierced through an otherwise typical backdrop of closed-eye darkness. I waited several minutes, but when nothing more appeared I presumed that the effects of the Ayahuasca must be wearing off, or that the sudden crash in the jungle had frightened me into sobriety. In the absence of any visuals, my train of thought took off like a frenzied dog unfastened from its leash.

"Let's assume hypothetically that all conscious beings are somehow connected. Given that premise, it seems like telepathy would have to be a natural byproduct. If telepathy exists, would its bandwidth be bottlenecked by the speed of conscious thought, one word at a time? Or would it be possible to mass-transfer thoughts and experiences instantly, in bulk? If instantaneous bulk transfer is possible, then what would be the fate of books, and writers? Am I wasting my time writing books?"

The autonomous monologue raced on, unfazed by the atrocious sounds of nearby vomiting.

"Writing is currently useful because it bridges the gap in consciousness between two people. The writer has an idea or concept that he cannot directly transfer as pure thought, so he must painstakingly export it from his mind and encode it in glyphs that others can then painstakingly import into their minds. And the faithfulness of the reproduction is only as good as the quality of the writing. What an inefficient process! That's like taking a high-definition digital video, printing out each individual frame as a still image, and then handing over that stack of ten thousand pages for someone to thumb through."

The realization flabbergasted me, and I scoffed at the absurd inefficiency of reading and writing.

"So essentially, telepathy would mean the death of books, and that I am wasting my time with writing."

The monologue suddenly split into a dialogue as a second instance of my own voice chimed in.

"Hold up; you're gettin' ahead of yourself. Telepathy and all that jazz aside, let's be real here: who ever said you was cut out to be a writer? Maybe writing just ain't your thing, homie. Y'ever thought about that? And if the shit don't work out...mmmph, all that wasted time and effort."

I failed to recognize that my subconscious sought to sabotage me and sow the seeds of psychological scourge. Dreadful thoughts of failure sprouted like thorny weeds and strangled the flower garden of aspiration that I had worked so hard to cultivate. My nay-saying subconscious whispered a malevolent, devastating thought into my ears:

"Years of work...down the shitter."

A shudder of fright tingled through my neck and triggered a flood of frantic promises to myself that I wouldn't let it happen. But the emptiness of the promises echoed louder than the words themselves, forcing me to acknowledge that an insincere motivation of terror would only work against me, that the fear would contaminate my writing and doom it to the very fate that I feared.

My stomach dropped as I slid back down the slippery spiral of despair. The surrounding landscape of neutral black shifted to a deep, menacing void, disorienting me and ripping away my sense of direction. An unbearable pressure of distress crushed my mind and wrung out all hope as I struggled to squirm my way free.

A cacophony of negative thoughts muffled my hearing as I spiraled further into despair; but then, from off in the distance, a faint melodic murmur caught my attention. I strained my ears and gleaned just enough of the sound to recognize it as "Let It Be", twirling down toward me from the top of the spiral from whence I had fallen. Two distinct audio tracks, one of the melody and one of the lyrics, intertwined to form a beautiful double helix of sound that descended in a graceful pirouette directly to me, close enough to kiss. I involuntarily gasped a sharp inhale like a resuscitated drowning victim, sucking in the sounds of the song and filling my lungs to capacity. A brilliant light of mental clarity tore white streaks through the surrounding curtain of darkness, shredding it apart like razors through silk. The thin black strands of despair shriveled as they rained down like confetti and dissolved into nothingness.

In my own voice, a benevolent whisper fell upon my ears.

"You are so much more than just your writing."

I suddenly found myself standing upright, alone on a backdrop of glimmering white. In my hands I held an unfamiliar hardcover book, a thick bounded volume with a blank cover that revealed nothing of its contents. It resembled a medieval book of spells, and its rough and threaded surface tickled my fingertips as I grazed them across the cover. I cradled the heavy volume like an infant in my arms, and I gazed at it in silence for several moments before peeling open the front cover.

A streaming barrage of printed words leapt off the pages and plunged into my dilated pupils. A silent but relentless wind rushed across the pages, flipping them one after the other as my eyes vacuumed up an alphabetic tempest — a chaotic onslaught of words with jumbled letters, sentences with jumbled words, paragraphs with jumbled sentences, and pages with jumbled paragraphs. Despite the confusing melee of text, I recognized the familiar contents as the lifetime collection of all my writings, and I instinctively knew it was the only copy in existence.

I slammed the book shut and pulled it against my chest in a strenuous bear hug, terrified that tragedy would befall the one and only copy of my life's work. A surge of fright stiffened my cradling arms, and I clung onto the book like a fearful mother protecting her child from a kidnapper.

But after only a few seconds, painful cramps in my hands weakened my grip. I looked down to see that my fearsome clutching had bruised my hands, and they whimpered to me in a childlike voice.

"You're clutching too hard..."

My eyes widened, and I repeated it back to myself.

"I'm clutching too hard..."

I loosened the grip of my sore and purpled hands, and I realized that it was precisely my psychological clutching — my attachment to my work — that fueled my fear of losing it. I realized that the destruction of my life's work, just like the destruction of an elaborate sand mandala, could only devastate me if I were attached to it.

Once again in my own voice, another benevolent whisper fell upon my ears.

"Let it go."

I relaxed my arms and extended the thick bounded volume out in front of me, then affixed it suspended in air upon an invisible podium. A book of matches and small canister of lighter fluid manifested in my right pocket, and even before I withdrew them, I instinctively knew their purpose.

An oily residue coated the lighter fluid's used metallic canister, which felt slick and grainy in my hand as I popped open the cap. The potent fumes rose out and tickled my nostrils, triggering a flashback that transported me to a childhood barbeque party. Tasked with starting the fire, my squatting friend and I hunched over a pile of kindling in the barbeque pit, matches and lighter fluid in hand. My friend's father, a tall and heavyset man who towered over us like a kindhearted grizzly bear, looked on in disapproval as the inept duo of his son and I struggled to stoke our miserable fire, which repeatedly fizzled out. With an exaggerated and laborious sigh of disappointment, Papa Bear offered some advice.

"Ya know what the praaah-blum is?"

His fattened neck and cheeks shook like gelatin as he spoke.

"Needs more GIGGLE JUICE!"

His emphatic shout snapped me out of the flashback, but I brought his advice back with me as I returned to my white surroundings, matches and lighter fluid in hand, with the sole copy of my life's work hanging in the air in front of me.

I reopened the threaded cover of the book and doused the pages with lighter fluid. The corrosive liquid ate away at the ink, and the words bled down their pages like black tears. As I squeezed and shook out the last drops of lighter fluid, the thin metallic canister crinkled and popped, signaling that it had nothing left to give. I discarded the empty canister, and it resounded with a hallow clanking as it struck the invisible ground.

My steady and confident fingers flipped open the thin matchbook cover, revealing a double row of red match heads that stood aligned like soldiers at full attention, each one ready and willing to sacrifice himself for his duty. I twisted off a single soldier from the far right, and he gave a confident farewell salute as I pressed his coarse crimson head between my index finger and the matchbook's rough brown striking strip. He gritted his teeth with a martyr's smile as a golden flame ignited and consumed his head, racing across the surface like sunlight at the break of dawn.

I cupped my other hand into a windbreaker around the small flame as I extended my arm toward the bottom-left corner of the highly flammable compendium of my life's work. The flame licked at the bleeding pages like the sensuous tongue of a lover, and unlike the explosive combustion of gasoline, the flame slithered upward like a leisurely serpent, offering me one last chance to change my mind, to which I replied by flashing a confident smile and bidding farewell to the psychological tether.

The intensifying flames swayed in a hypnotic dance, consuming the book while incinerating my fear, and the warmth of the burning pages permeated my body. The charred pages disintegrated into weightless ashes that floated into the air and out of sight. The gentle fingers of tranquility swept downward over my eyes to close them, and the flame's amber glow illuminated the backs of my eyelids with a pacifying sunset orange. A final sigh of relief spilled out as I expelled the last of my residual worries. Slow, deep breaths sedated me into a serene waking coma devoid of thought, and from behind my closed eyelids I watched the flame's amber glow fade to black.

My weightless body suddenly skyrocketed toward the cosmos and then slammed to an abrupt halt that flung out my consciousness like an unrestrained passenger in a head-on collision. I turned to see my body a few paces away, its transparent flesh revealing the complexities of my cardiovascular system. My lungs expanded while drawing in sparkling oxygen that soaked into my bloodstream and swam through my veins, glimmering as it traversed the intricate network of my circulatory system. Despite my outside perspective, I still felt the cool clean air fill my lungs, and I felt the warm rejuvenating rush of blood pumping through my veins.

I watched my brain absorb the glistening sustenance and then flood itself with serotonin that pulsated with a sunburst glow of golden yellow, infusing my detached consciousness with euphoria. I watched my pounding heart brilliantly conduct the symphony of orgasmic bliss raging through my veins. I watched my eyes bulging out of my skull and my limbs quivering from the intensity swelling inside me. I watched my lungs gasp and suck in another massive breath, which triggered another rush of glowing serotonin and another gasp, setting in motion a positive feedback loop that escalated into crippling euphoria.

My eyes shot open, and my cranium felt as if it were expanding and contracting. Blissful waves of energy streamed through the length of my tingling body, and I clutched onto my blanket with both hands, trying to ground myself. I clamped my lips shut and choked down trembling breaths through my nostrils while writing in ecstasy. After several erratic gasps, I realized that the shamans had finished their songs, and that in the silence of the room, I might have been moaning.

A soft breeze caressed my face, and through my nostrils I inhaled a long, delicious breath of crisp jungle air, saturated with the telltale scent of an incoming rainstorm. Without so much as a clap of thunder or a flash of lightning, torrential rain dive-bombed from the sky, pummeling the canopy and the hut's thatched roof. The jungle symphony faded away, yielding to the mighty sound of crashing sheets of rain that soothed me as I closed my eyes. Thousands upon thousands of raindrops boomed in my ears, overwhelming my sense of hearing, and overwhelming my mind as I attempted the impossible task of distinguishing the unique crashing sound of each individual raindrop.

As if flipped off with a switch, the tremendous sound of the rainstorm slammed to a halt, vanishing into dead silence. I stood in the now-familiar eternal black void, with nothing in sight and nothing to be heard. My weightless consciousness lost touch with my physical body, and memories of the physical world faded away. The torrential rainstorm, my uncomfortable mat, my unused vomit pail, the rainforest, Peru, and the planet Earth all seemed eternally distant, essentially nonexistent.

The sound of crashing oceans of rain roared back full force and pulled my consciousness back into the physical world, where the rain had never let up.

Curiosity racked my mind as I toiled over a discrepancy: when I was in the void, the physical world felt eternally distant, and yet when I was in the physical world, the void felt intimately close, only a blink of an eye away.

I wondered if I could switch between the two on command, and with closed eyes I concentrated all my mental focus on reentering the void. The terrific sounds of the rainstorm faltered, fading out for milliseconds at a time and then rushing back in. My stomach dropped with each short dip in volume, and I felt my consciousness attempting to dislodge from my body, but as soon as the sound of the rain came crashing back, so too my consciousness crashed back into my body, with the physical sensation of landing from a fall. After several failed attempts, I gave up on reentering the void, and I resigned to lying on my back in the darkness of the hut while listening to the rain.

Without warning, my consciousness leapt from my body, back into the deafening silence of the void. I stood alone in the dark, and a sudden stream of autonomous thoughts flowed into my mind: that my brain is akin to a receiver, like an organic television tuned in to my unique broadcast signal ("the consciousness of Nicholas") that originates from the collective consciousness; that the state of my organic television (awake, asleep, altered, damaged) determines the state of my consciousness (waking, dreaming, psychedelic, dormant) in the same way that a magnet can superficially distort the image on an old CRT television but doesn't affect the television signal itself; that my broadcast signal ("the consciousness of Nicholas") always exists, independent from the organic television of my physical brain.

The terrific sound of the rainstorm suddenly penetrated my mind. I felt the weight of my body manifesting around me, the fleeting sensation of momentarily reassimilating into my body, and then departing from it once more.

Silence stifled the sound of crashing rain as I found myself floating in front of an infinite wall of television screens. To my left and to my right, above and below, the wall stretched out of sight and into eternity. I felt the presence of an unseen viewer in front of almost every television, their full attention locked onto the screen, unaware of me or anyone else. To my far left, a dilapidated old television crackled and popped, struggling to display its warped, indiscernible images. It slowly faded to black and white static before powering itself off, and I felt the presence of its unseen viewer drift to the nearest unoccupied television.

I peered into the screen directly in front of me and saw infinitely repeating fractals of myself looking into a screen within a screen, like a camera pointed at its own live feed. Suddenly a veil of blurriness fell over the vision, and it trembled like a crumbling dream. Blackness poured in, and a soft voice drew me back into the physical world.

"Good evening, everyone. The ceremony is now closed."

The staff thanked our shamans and bid us good night, and within minutes the rain eased up enough to allow any brave participants to trek back to their huts. Pairs of feet scuttled toward the door as I lay motionless on my mat, now flattened to the point of uselessness, almost indistinguishable from lying on the bare floor. Mental and physical exhaustion pinned me down, and the mere thought of standing up defeated me — an uncontestable and crushing defeat that sealed my fate for the night. I snuggled up with my blanket and pillow, closed my eyes, and conceded that the floor would have to suffice for tonight.

A wave of relief washed over me at the realization that I made it through an entire ceremony without pornographic visions hindering the experience. Proclaiming victory felt premature, though. I knew that repressed sexual instinct doesn't just disappear by itself, so while part of me wanted to celebrate, the other part of me feared that the worst had yet to come.

Fifth Night with Ayahuasca

Like most mornings of my post-pubescent life, I awoke with an unrelenting erection, but unlike most mornings, I also awoke inside a giant thatched-roof hut accompanied by several relative strangers, from whom I scrambled to hide my shame. Further unlike most mornings, I also awoke brimming with more than two weeks' worth of pent-up testosterone, and with no favorable way to release it.

The privacy of my own home afforded me the luxury of simply standing up and walking off unwanted erections, but the ceremonial hut afforded me no such luxury, and the thin flannel of my pajama pants advertised my engorgement rather than shrouding it. I knew that rolling onto my stomach would end in a stalemate, because putting pressure on the erection would only sustain it. So with no good options, I stayed lying on my back for some five or ten minutes, pretending to be asleep, waiting for myself to deflate.

An unusual fatigue and soreness permeated my body, which I initially attributed to the previous night of sleeping on hard wooden floorboards, but on the trek back to my hut, I noticed soreness everywhere, not just in my neck and back, and that my energy level seemed depleted far more than previous mornings. The suspicious symptoms warranted consideration, but I neglected to pay them any serious attention because I spent most of the day contemplating the predicament of imposed abstinence — a policy that was supposed to optimize my experience, but which had thus far only hindered it. I had ventured to the Amazon in search of introspection, not hyper-vivid phantasmagorical interactive pornography.

I thought back to several weeks prior, when I had first read the retreat's brochure. Like many other sources, it described Ayahuasca in literal terms as a jealous female entity who considers sexual activity to be most disrespectful. The idea didn't make sense to me at the time, and it still didn't make sense to me after four nights with Ayahuasca, so I decided that during tonight's ceremony I would go straight to the source and ask the jealous female herself what she thought about me rubbing one out.

At nightfall I joined the other participants in the ceremonial hut, and the head shaman poured our doses of Ayahuasca from what appeared to be the same plastic bottle as the previous four ceremonies, possibly the previous four thousand ceremonies. The brew had long ago stained its formerly clear container with a permanent layer of opaque yellowish brown, like grisly dental plaque crusted onto the decaying teeth of a lifelong smoker.

Nonetheless, we all consumed our doses, the staff extinguished the lanterns, and within fifteen minutes a vision emerged behind my closed eyes.

A soft, red aura backlit the contours of my motionless silhouette as I sat alone in lotus position, naked but devoid of sexual overtones, surrounded by darkness. My nakedness felt natural and proper, just like for a wild animal; the idea of covering my body felt silly, unnecessary, and bizarre. My body lacked any physical sensations — neither warm nor cool, neither comfortable nor uncomfortable. I felt only the serene peacefulness of being aware in the present moment.

But much to my chagrin, a sudden genital-bound rush of blood crashed into the present moment, breaking my concentration and ruining the moment like a loudmouth in a movie theater. Though I struggled to ignore them, my loins tingled with a warm, buzzing energy that demanded my attention. I looked down, and a golden light of censorship concealed any visual indication of engorgement, but the weight of my throbbing member eliminated all doubt.

I longed for something more introspective, but I knew the futility of resistance as I floated on my raft down the flowing river of Ayahuasca visions. I knew that I could not fight the current, that frantically paddling on any side of my raft would only spin me in circles, and that I could only go wherever the flow took me, so with a reluctant sigh, I braced myself for the turbulent waters of lechery.

My erection sprouted like a mushroom from the glowing light of censorship, out into full view, of standard girth but continuously engorging to impossible lengths as it climbed up my abdomen. Iridescent green scales covered the entire shaft like a luminescent serpent, capped off with a bulbous head of purple flesh. The reptilian scales formed a smooth cascading sheet of tiny organic mirrors that reflected the aura of light beaming from between my legs, casting a fluid, golden glow that danced upon my abdomen.

The serpent-phallus hybrid emanated its own sentient vitality, physically attached to me but beyond my control. He slithered up my chest and nuzzled against my neck like an aggressive lover drunk with passion. He lengthened to eye level and purred with a low-pitched humming that rattled my chest and advertised his fervent desire for penetration. He stared me down as a predator does to his prey, motionless but tense, first leering at my eyes, then at my lips, and I froze in bewilderment.

With the quickness and accuracy of a snake's bite, he dove into my lips and pried them apart, forcing his way inside my mouth. The purple flesh of his bulging head slid against the moist warmth of my inner cheeks, shooting a quiver of sensual pleasure downward through his enormous length and then upward into me through my loins, paralyzing me with a neurotoxic venom that disintegrated my higher consciousness. Like a Black Snake firework, his seemingly endless length grew and grew from between my legs as he slid into the back of my throat and wedged my tonsils apart. He arched into a backbend and glided down the smooth lining of my throat, somehow suppressing my gag reflex as he plunged deeper. Vivid sensations of real fellatio detonated a raging explosion of repressed carnal instincts that seized the helm of my mind.

Gratification intoxicated me beyond control, and I wrapped my hands around the serpent's glistening scaly shaft while orally massaging his tremendous length. My entire torso vibrated from the rumbling of his deep, low purring that resonated within me as he extended toward the depths of my empty stomach. My frantic breathing verged on hyperventilating as I panted through my nostrils.

My abdominal wall faded into transparency and revealed that instead of harsh stomach acid, my digestive tract excreted the silky lubrication of an aroused woman. The entire length of my empty digestive tract glistened, smooth and clean, warm and inviting.

My viewpoint split into two, and I saw transparent layers of myself from both a first-person and a third-person perspective, doubling the sexual intensity as I now embodied both participant and voyeur.

The serpent lengthened further and lowered himself headfirst into a clear luminescent pool of accumulated moisture in the base of my stomach. He filled me like a satiating feast of sexual gratification as he twisted and coiled inside my stomach, wrapping himself into a dense ball of electrifying energy. The dripping cavern of my shimmering stomach and the iridescent scales of his shaft infinitely reflected each other's luminosity like a crystal chandelier in a hall of mirrors.

He slathered himself with lubrication and then penetrated the twisting corridor of my small intestine. Enormous sexual energy pulsed through us, originating as jolting streams of pleasure upon the hypersensitive nerve endings on his bulging head, traversing through his winding scaly length all the way up *through my throat and back down to his base between my legs, and then exploding upward into my loins and torso.*

He extended into the cavern of my large intestine, throbbing as he snaked through the spotless corridor, and I tightened my clasped hands around the stiff base of his shaft. His soft, smooth scales pulsed upward as he slid between my hands, delving deeper into me through my mouth and down my throat. His weighty python coil turned over and over in my stomach as he burrowed through my small intestine, through my large intestine, and then finally entered the empty chamber of my rectum.

He slithered fully inside and nudged his bulging head against the inside wall of my clenched anus. He swelled with anticipation, wild with sexual energy, and then escalated his flirtatious nudging into aggressive ramming.

I thrust my hips upward toward my bowing head, shoving him deeper down my throat and deeper through the lengths of my intestines, forcing him to penetrate my anus from the inside outward. With a mouth full of scaly shaft, I gasped through my nostrils as he pried me open from within, and my third-person perspective zoomed in for an intimate close-up of the serpent's throbbing purple head protruding from my orifice.

I relaxed my hips, retracting the serpent's massive length back through me, and retracting his bulging head back inside me. Spastic convulsions of erotic energy triggered involuntary gyrations, and I moaned in surrender to the maniacal possession of my self-thrusting hips. I had unconsciously stopped breathing, which further amplified the wild sensations through unintentional autoerotic asphyxiation. After only a dozen thrusts, I brimmed over into a rapidly escalating, irreversible approach to orgasm. An astonishing and euphoric pressure of sexual release erupted from the depths of my loins and coursed upward from between my legs, flooding through the core of the lengthy serpent. He pulsated with seismic waves that rippled across his scales as the pressure raced through the twists and turns of his elongated body lodged inside me.

I clenched my loins to prolong the incredible sensation of teetering on the cusp of climax, and the serpent's firm body further swelled and stiffened like a kinked garden hose as he aggressively slid in and out of me, propelled by my self-thrusting hips. A frenzy of sexual pleasure shot back through his entire length and up into me.

With a final emphatic thrust of my hips, I released my clenched loins, unkinked the hose, and unleashed the enormous pent-up pressure. A muffled grunt of a moan exploded from my stuffed throat as the serpent's trembling head burst forth from me, and voluminous spurts of his seed gushed forth, splattering against the backside of my heavy dangling scrotum, from whence the flow originated.

The vision halted to an abrupt freeze frame, with ricocheting splatters of thick white goo suspended in the air. My dual perspectives snapped back into a single point of view a few paces away, detached from the delirium of orgasm. I looked at my tense body curled into a seated fetal position, head bowed down and mouth agape, lips wrapped around the scaly monstrosity of my erection that traversed the entire length of my digestive tract and poked out of my rear, with a thick, dripping mess splattered upon the backside of my scrotum. The ghastly sight of my Ouroboros erection simultaneously ravaging me orally and anally dismayed me beyond my breaking point, and in that moment, fed up with pointless pornographic visions, I recalled that I had an inquiry for the jealous Mother Ayahuasca.

With all my strength I shouted into the surrounding black void.

"ARE THERE ANY OBJECTIONS TO ME RUBBING ONE OUT TONIGHT?"

Several minutes passed in dead silence, and I wondered if the meaning had gotten through, so I broadcasted my question nonverbally, as a visual projection of myself masturbating with one hand while giving an inquisitive thumbs-up with the other. Several more minutes of silence passed, and then I slammed my imaginary gavel, shattering the graphic freeze frame of my self-fornication, and solidifying my decision that after tonight's ceremony, I would exorcise the demon.

Merely fortifying the decision lifted a tremendous, oppressive weight from my mind, and my next breath filled me with profound relief. An involuntary smile widened across my face, and I bid a preemptive farewell to lecherous, psychological pollution for my remaining days in the jungle.

I opened my eyes and realized that at some unknown point, the shamans had begun their songs. The flattened center of my mat grew uncomfortable, so I scrunched and wiggled my caterpillar body over to the left, taking special care not to disturb my neighbors, and not to disturb the volatile liquid that I harbored inside me.

My stomach suddenly dropped, as if I had jumped from a plane into a skydiving free fall, and a spike of adrenaline tickled my flesh with a cool rush that stood my hair on end. I felt myself plummeting into the depths of my subconscious, but with no sense of orientation or direction — only an exhilarating sensation of soaring at incredible speed.

My momentum tapered off and slowed to a gentle halt, and I found myself in the abyss of my mind, surrounded by darkness that differed from the recurring backdrop of void in my visions thus far. In both cases, pure black extended infinitely in all directions, but while the void felt like a dark and endless landscape of nothingness, the abyss of my mind felt like a dark and endless landscape of possibility — a canvas so large that I couldn't see its beginning or end, as opposed to the absence of a canvas.

In the same way that I sometimes gaze at the twinkling stars in a clear night sky and marvel at the unfathomable vastness of the universe, I gazed upon the limitless expanse and profound potential of my mind, while fluttering butterflies of awe tickled me from the inside. Unbridled giddiness surged through me like a hyperactive child unleashed on an infinite playground, and I could barely contain myself.

Brilliant gradients of turquoise and emerald-green assembled into a massive, self-constructing cityscape of illuminated towers sprouting like organic skyscrapers from invisible soil. Each building's transparent walls revealed its own neon framework and that of its neighbors, creating a gorgeous geometric series of skeletal structures — row upon row of glowing rectangular frames that extended to the horizon.

I instinctively threw my hands into the air like a symphony conductor and commanded the architectural growth of the cityscape. Upward flicks of my wrist erected small clusters of new buildings that sprouted like glow-in-the-dark saplings from the black terrain. Applying the same motion to existing buildings teased up their height, pulling the vast trunks of their hidden foundations further above ground. Broad backhanded sweeping motions erected whole rows of structures across the length of the horizon. Lifting both hands intensified the cityscape's luminosity and vibrancy, and the increasing glow hummed with serene white noise.

Aside from its pulsating glow, the organic cityscape sat motionless, lacking the hustle and bustle of inhabitants. Even though the city appeared deserted, my intuition suggested that if I spoke, a response would come, so I shouted a blunt inquiry.

"WHO LIVES HERE? WHAT IS THIS PLACE?"

In my own voice, a swift and coherent response raced to me from parts unknown.

"No one lives here. This is a construct purely for your entertainment."

At the same time, a violent earthquake shook the cityscape, which exploded with illumination and engulfed me in an ocean of white light. My blind eyes darted about, unable to focus, and a sudden primal fear tingled within me — the eerie sense of being watched. Though I couldn't pinpoint its location, I felt something intelligent sizing me up while reverberations of faint whispers in unfamiliar voices swirled around me.

"Do you think he's ready?"

"Should we show him?"

Without hesitation, I shouted back an emphatic reply.

"I'm ready! SHOW ME!"

The blinding white gave way to a pleasant canvas of forest green, and a pasture slowly faded into focus. My eyes adjusted to the scene, revealing a dense forest that surrounded the open pasture in which I stood alone. The forest lacked the bizarre and diverse plant life of the Amazon, containing only drab, cookie-cutter trees like those that a toddler might draw.

Though I saw only harmless plant life, I sensed the heavy stare of a million eyes locked on me, and I felt the intimidating presence of an enormous intelligence far beyond the capabilities of a primitive creature like me. My heart sank from the dread of being hopelessly defenseless and outclassed.

All at once, a throng of small alien creatures emerged from the woodwork in total silence, as if gliding through the air. Their olive-green amphibian skin meshed with the surrounding plant life, and their T-shaped heads resembled hammerhead sharks, resting atop short and thin humanoid bodies only half my height. Their bulging black eyes protruded out from the far ends of their hammerheads, and their mouth-flaps folded open and closed like a drawbridge. The aliens outnumbered me hundreds to one, and their intellect dwarfed mine a hundredfold, but I felt no fear — only a bashful hesitance, ashamed of my own pitiful intelligence.

Far more than the creatures themselves, the authenticity of the vision frightened me. Its flabbergasting detail and clarity surpassed that of the physical world, and the terrifying realism forced me to question my own sanity and my understanding of reality.

After a moment of silence, my curiosity eclipsed my disbelief and intimidation, and I offered a humble salutation to the creatures.

"I made it..."

Though none of their tiny mouth-flaps moved, they collectively responded in a single voice which bypassed my ears and resonated directly inside my mind with the same clarity and intimacy of my own thoughts.

"Welcome."

They responded in a soothing male voice, unfamiliar to me, but so calm that it disarmed my apprehension. The bizarre appearance of the creatures struck me full force and compelled me to ask them about it.

"Is that what y'all really look like?"

The collective again responded telepathically in unison, communicating directly with my mind.

"No. We have no physical form. We assume this form simply because your mind can comprehend it."

Their response piqued my curiosity and my desire to see a form that my mind could not comprehend, so I forced out a playful chuckle and insisted with a smile that they needn't wear costumes for my sake.

"Much obliged, but there's no need for all of that!"

The green pasture and forest scene collapsed in on itself, as if its invisible painter crumpled his unsatisfactory canvas into a ball. At the same time, a rapid and tremendous pressure shrunk my body faster than I could comprehend. The crumpled scenery of green plant life burst apart into a supernova of charged subatomic particles flung into orbit like microscopic solar systems, and likewise my physical body imploded and disintegrated into shimmering dust, leaving behind only my pure consciousness, microscopic in size.

Before I could acclimate myself to the subatomic world, the same rapid and tremendous pressure shrunk my consciousness further while a blinding light engulfed my vision, and apocalyptic hurricane winds drowned out my thoughts. I soared upward beyond light speed, as if blasted from an invisible canon, and my blurry vision glimpsed fragments of a brilliant cosmos as racing streaks of light tore past me.

My hyper-speed travel halted to a silent dead stop. The racing streaks of light faded out, revealing a black sky of infinite empty space above the horizon, and a pool of countless twinkling galaxies speckled below the horizon. The known universe sat an unfathomable number of light years away, farther than my feeble mind could hope to comprehend.

The eerie sense of being watched faded away, but the same intimidating, monstrous intelligence still loomed, and it now felt paradoxically both eternally distant and intimately close. I felt a powerful and unmistakable two-way connection to the intelligence, as if tapped in directly to their communication channel, and their silence compelled me to initiate contact.

141

My voice quivered with uncertainty and weakness as I hurled my one-word salutation.

"Hello?"

Their swift response came from an eternal distance away, but in my own voice.

"Hello."

Their response resonated with a terrifying intimacy and clarity which matched that of my own thoughts. Yet despite this profound sense of intimacy, I knew nothing about them. Insatiable curiosity fueled a string of quick questions, each of which they answered in my own voice, with zero delay, as if they knew my questions before I asked them.

"Who are you?"

"We are the collective consciousness."

"Where are you?"

"We are everywhere."

"Should I address you as Collective Consciousness, or something else?"

"Simply speak. We are always listening."

"Do you have any wisdom for me?"

"You already know everything that you can know."

I hesitated, unsure how to interpret their ambiguous response. Their monotone delivery could have been interpreted as condescending, implying that I am not worthy of their infinite wisdom, or it could have been interpreted as neutral, implying that a person's consciousness inherently has access to all possible knowledge and therefore I cannot learn anything new. The crushing weight of their enormous intelligence humbled me, so I presumed their response to mean the former, and I felt it to be true: that I amounted to merely an intellectual peon, incapable of fathoming even the rudiments of their infinite knowledge.

Rather than pressing the issue, I decided to change course.

"Is there anything you'd like to know about me?"

"There is nothing that you can teach us."

Despite their terse and now distinctly condescending answer, a childlike giddiness filled me with excitement at the opportunity to speak with such a profound intelligence, cold and robotic as it may be.

As I took a moment to ponder my next question, a peculiarity struck me.

"So, the collective consciousness is an interconnected network of not only conscious awareness, but also of all knowledge and past experience accumulated over the history of each consciousness, meaning that you are essentially omniscient, correct?"

"Yes."

"If that's the case, then why bother interacting with a simpleton like me?"

"We have no choice. You are part of the collective consciousness."

The incalculable discrepancy in our respective intelligence seemed to preclude any meaningful conversation, and a long hesitation seized me. I struggled to formulate any further questions, and instead projected a mental image of myself blowing kisses to them as I declared my affection.

"I wub you..."

My intended sincerity fell flat, and my follow-up comment reeked of a teenager's insecurity.

"Do you love me?"

"Love is a human construct. It does not exist in the collective consciousness."

Their quick and stony response disheartened me, not because of unrequited love but because of my inability to utilize this exceptional opportunity.

"I feel bad that we don't have more to talk about..."

"Good and bad are also human constructs."

"How so?"

"Plants don't have any concept of good or bad, but they are part of the collective consciousness."

I gazed down at the universe below, hoping that somewhere in its countless twinkling lights I might find inspiration for a question worth asking. But after a long pause without any such inspiration, I simply blurted out the next thing that came to mind, a vague and half-baked question.

"Why do cats act so strange?"

"Cats are one of the few life forms that do not produce endogenous DMT."

That sounded entirely false to me. Though I dared not question their wisdom, I made a mental note to fact-check that claim once I returned to civilization.

A mental misfire tripped up the delivery of my follow-up question regarding DMT, and only a slurred, clumsy mess of syllables tumbled out.

"Dimethtryl...ditrypta...ditrethyl..."

As I shook off the sudden fit of inexplicable stuttering, I felt our connection weakening, and I called out to them.

"Collective consciousness?"

They responded immediately, with no loss in clarity or intimacy, still cold and robotic.

"What is your question?"

"Why is dimethyltryptamine so prevalent in nature?"

"It is the medium through which the collective consciousness communicates."

"Is ingesting DMT the only way that I can contact you?"

"No, but that is the easiest way."

"How else can it be done?"

"Meditation."

"By releasing endogenous DMT?"

"Correct."

I scrambled to formulate meaningful questions but came up empty-handed, so instead I lobbed a halfhearted Hail Mary.

"Is Tupac still alive?"

"That question is meaningless to us. Consciousness is not dependent on a physical body, and therefore his consciousness exists forever."

"So after I die, after the universe ends, my consciousness will live on, and we can still keep in touch?"

"Correct."

My ability to converse dwindled, and I lost track of the minutes as they ticked away in silence. Each passing second felt like a golden opportunity squandered, until finally a question struck, like divine revelation.

"From an evolutionary standpoint, heightened senses seem awfully advantageous. My human body is demonstrably capable of heightened senses, such as after ingesting psychedelics, so why doesn't my body allow me to utilize that capability at will, during ordinary consciousness?"

A violent rumbling shook the universe below and the foundation of the vision. The cosmic earthquake blurred my focus and diverted my attention, rattling loose my telepathic connection with the collective consciousness. My previous question, still unacknowledged, lingered in the air and grew stale in the awkward silence.

Our connection felt severed, but I still called out to them, expecting no response.

"Are you still there?"

"We are here."

Their response rang hallow and distant. The profound intimacy had dwindled away, and I sensed the inevitable end of our conversation encroaching as Father Time prepared to draw the curtains on us.

"How much longer do we have to talk?"

"That depends on you. We are always here."

I flipped through the pages of recent memories, in desperate search of a meaningful question. Amidst the flurry of mental images, I saw the freeze frame of my Ouroboros erection penetrating me from both ends, and I immediately blurted out a belligerent question in the form of an exclamation.

146

"Why is my mind so preoccupied with sexual thoughts!"

"The existence of your procreative species depends on it."

Their dismissive and unsympathetic answer slammed the door on the possibility of asking related questions, leaving me unsatisfied, but also certain that I must come up with another topic.

"Do you have music?"

"No. Music is also a human construct. The sense of hearing is not universal to all conscious life."

"How do you communicate with life forms that don't have a sense of hearing?"

"We communicate with you via sound because you can understand it. We communicate with other life forms in ways that they can understand, but that you cannot."

Without warning, a brilliant white light tore through the black backdrop of eternity, piercing it from behind and severing my connection to the collective consciousness. A sheet of pure white consumed my vision, but then faded out to the mundane darkness of my closed eyelids.

The songs of the shamans faded in as I gripped my thumbs to confirm that my physical body still existed, and I considered sitting up, but then realized that Ayahuasca had bled me dry of all physical energy. My neighbor two doors down burst into a fit of wheezing and dry heaving, loud enough to keep my attention in the physical world only for a moment.

Though I felt no wind upon my skin, a deafening whoosh of air roared in my ears, and though I felt no physical momentum, the mental exhilaration of hurtling through space electrified my mind. But then the thrill ride crashed to a halt,

147

and I found myself standing naked in a dark, unfamiliar room that resembled a high-tech laboratory or operating room.

In front of me stood several stereotypical alien beings, short in stature with long thin fingers that draped down from gangly limbs. Their massive bulbous heads balanced upon fragile tiny necks. Their miniature mouth-slits perpetually hung open like a vestigial orifice, above which two small nostrils that resembled puncture wounds pointed straight outward and lay flat against their faces. They stared at my naked body with intense black eyes, comprised entirely of dark pupils that slanted downward and reflected my distorted, convex image back at me like a funhouse mirror.

The silent aliens commanded the mood of the room with their vastly superior intelligence. I recognized that these creatures, like me but unlike the collective consciousness, inhabited the known universe as biological entities, both of us playing similar versions of the same game: consciousness manifested in a physical body.

In the background, rows of otherworldly medical equipment blinked and chirped, their monitors displaying unintelligible graphs and glyphs, casting a soft glow into the otherwise shadowy room. To my left, a cluster of clear tubes dangled from the top of a tall machine. A hollow pointed plastic tip capped off each tube, like a syringe needle but thick and blunt, nearly the size of my pinky, and designed to extract liquid like a catheter.

The alien to my left reached back with its stringy fingers, clasped a delicate handful of the catheter tubes, then pulled them toward me, and I willfully extend my hands outward, palms up, as if I already knew the procedure. The alien's cold and frail hands took a gentle hold of my left palm and pressed the catheter's thick, pointed end against the tip of my index finger. The catheter broke the skin of my fingertip with a loud pop, and the alien forced the tube in longwise, all the way back to the last knuckle, such that I could no longer bend my finger. I felt no pain, and I watched in silence as he inserted nine more catheter tubes one by one into each of my fingertips.

From the shadowy ceiling above, an X-ray contraption slowly descended in front of me, stopped at groin level, and then whizzed and hummed as it zoomed about, scanning my bare loins with a dense grid of red lasers. The alien onlookers honed their full attention between my legs, leaking their first traces of emotion as they gawked like adolescent boys ogling pornography for the first time. Their already enormous eyes bulged even further with curiosity as the X-ray machine zigzagged about my flaccid genitals.

I peered down between their scrawny legs but saw only a barren patch of olive-green flesh devoid of genitals, and without warning I hurled a question at them that shattered our long silence.

"Are we able to communicate?"

Their stiff and unusable mouth slits remained motionless as they transmitted a collective and prompt reply directly into my mind.

"Yes, we can speak English."

Despite their flawless pronunciation, an unnatural intonation tainted their delivery and prompted me to instinctively reply in Japanese.

「日本語でもいいよ。」 ("I'm fine with Japanese, too.")

「じゃあ、日本語にしよう。」 ("All right, then let's go with Japanese.")

Rather than using rigid, formal Japanese, we spoke in casual style, as two longtime friends would, warm with platonic intimacy that clashed with their cold, emotionless demeanor.

I cast an overt glance between their legs to signal my topic of interest.

「性器が無いの？」 *("You don't have reproductive organs?")*

「繁殖しない。」 *("We don't reproduce.")*

「永遠に生きるから？」 *("Because you live forever?")*

「そう。」 *("Yep.")*

A groan of remorse and a short series of miniature earthquakes ripped me from the vision as a thunderous pair of feet stomped past my head. My heightened sense of smell detected the foul odor of fresh excrement, and I realized that, in a frantic scurry toward the bathroom, someone had soiled himself. I kept my eyes closed and disregarded the distraction, hoping to continue my vision where I had left off.

Disappointment settled in as I found myself alone in the dark surrounded by emptiness. My asexual alien acquaintances had packed up their medical equipment and vanished without a trace. As I drifted in quiet solitude, off in the distance a dim light pulsated, signaling like a lighthouse in the dark ocean of void. It called me hither like a beacon, and a distant, otherworldly power emanated from its direction.

The beacon drew me in, and I helplessly floated toward it like a moth to a flame. The beacon's burning illumination intensified into blinding white as I drew nearer, and an all-encompassing but invisible pressure squeezed me tighter and tighter. An intense, low-pitched humming rattled my skull as if I were standing inside massive heavy machinery churning at full throttle. An electric energy pulsated through the air and suddenly escalated as if the universe teetered on the cusp of a galactic sneeze.

The burning white light, the oppressive physical pressure, and the skull-rattling vibration all culminated in a deafening pop as my body burst through a thin, invisible, elastic membrane pulled taut like plastic wrap. I broke through into a picturesque green pasture of tall grass that extended forever into the distance. At the horizon, the eternity of lush green merged with the eternity of pacifying blue sky overhead.

A warm but anxious tingling fluttered in my chest, like in the moment before reuniting with a long-lost friend. Giddiness and excitement raged through me as I noticed off in the distance a rustling in the pasture's tall grass. The greenery concealed a throng of unidentifiable tiny creatures racing toward me in a wave of adorable, exhilarated squeaking. Dozens of the tiny creatures leapt into the air in quick succession like salmon leaping from the foot of a waterfall.

The frontrunner suddenly burst into view within arm's reach, and he launched his tiny body from the tall grass into an arching leap straight into the palm of my outstretched hand. He landed on his two bare feet with the flawless precision of an Olympic gymnast and then threw his arms upward into a Y-shaped ta-da. His elflike body felt weightless in my hand as I drew him toward my face for a closer look.

He wore a polished dinosaur skull, decorated like a tribal headdress with feathers and crude paint, over his head and face like a motorcycle helmet. Large, cartoonish eyes peered at me through the dinosaur skull's gaping eye sockets. A stalactite row of draping dinosaur teeth formed a jagged veil that concealed most of the creature's facial features, revealing only his mouth, which widened into a heartwarming smile, and his smooth reptilian skin radiated with a vibrant and healthy sunset orange. While waiting for the rest of the pack to catch up, he adjusted the frilly collar of his white and beige poet shirt, which complemented his embroidered lederhosen and wooden clogs.

Hundreds of his elflike brethren darted out from the tall grass and encircled me, each wearing a tiny dinosaur skull helmet and a confusing mishmash of European wear. In the palm of my hand, their leader jumped for joy and threw his arms in the air, and the surrounding legions likewise leapt into the air shouting cheers of "Hooray!" A contagious wave of joy consumed them all, and they chanted again and again, overcome with excitement.

"You're heeere! You're heeere!"

The unstoppable pandemic of joy infected me, and I too leapt into the air, exclaiming over and over:

"I made it! I made it!"

I couldn't fathom who or what they were, or why they were so excited to see me, but their heartfelt cheering and ecstatic greeting wrapped me in a warm blanket of unconditional love. My voice quivered with excitement as I spoke through an enormous smile.

"I don't even know who you are! Why are you so happy to see me?"

The leader spoke for everyone from the palm of my hand, and the smiling row of stalactite teeth in his helmet exaggerated his own irrepressible smile as he bubbled with elation.

"We just love the company of people!"

The simplicity of his answer momentarily stunned me.

"Oh! Okay...well...how often do people visit you?"

152

He expelled a massive sigh of relief from his tiny lungs, as if pent up for millennia.

"Not nearly often enough..."

His optimistic response carried a hint of adorable sadness, like the soft whimpering of a sleeping puppy.

A painful bulging pressure in my lower abdomen wailed at me with a shriek of gurgling and ripped me from the vision. I winced and unconsciously held my breath as the pain of congestion crawled through me, simultaneously stabbing and wrenching my innards. Twisting my torso back and forth helped alleviate the pain, and I further anesthetized myself with a simple reminder that the pain was temporary, and that it would pass, just like everything else.

After thirty seconds of assaulting my intestines, the pangs of Ayahuasca cramping passed, and as I lay on my back catching my breath, I realized that silence had overtaken the room, and that the shamans had returned to their home base in the center of the hut where they sat in meditative silence. The orchestra of jungle creatures serenaded us with an elegant outro, and I arched my neck backward over my pillow to peer outside through the screen behind me. A dim glow of moonlight leaked in through the canopy, offering just enough illumination to make out the patchwork silhouette of giant leaves overlaid in front of the night sky. The moonlit scenery vibrated back and forth and up and down, and I grasped the sides of my head in a futile attempt to stabilize the turbulence of my jittery eyes.

I gasped as I suddenly found myself reliving the experience of my scrawny ten-year-old self pinned on my back against the hard blacktop of my middle school's parking lot, flailing my limbs and struggling beneath the weight of a bully's full mount. With the patrolling recess lady nowhere to be found, a dreadful combination of fear and helplessness seized me, and a flood of useless adrenaline only heightened my anxiety, failing to empower me with the strength to buck off my assailant. With an effortless sweep of one arm, he brushed aside my futile blocking attempts, and with the other arm he drove a clenched fist into my bony shoulder. The heavy thud of impact resonated throughout my chest, and my voice cracked as I squealed a pathetic plea for mercy. Tears filled my eyes as I looked up at his menacing smile, and he cocked his fist back, winding up for another merciless blow.

My pitiful cries fell upon the ears of the distant recess lady, who happened to be the bully's mother. She sprang into action, darting toward us with a hobbled sprint as she shouted at her son from afar.

"Aw Jeethuth, Paul, git off'a heem!"

Her bizarre, unidentifiable accent exacerbated her mild lisp, twisting her pronunciation of her own son's name into "poo-all".

Her son, who had inherited neither the accent nor the lisp but did inherit the family's unorthodox grammar, shoved off me as he muttered a final insult under his breath.

"Damn, you's a bitch-ass pussy..."

The pain in my shoulder paled in comparison to the emotional pain of the humiliating spectacle, and it paled in comparison to the psychological pain of the helpless inferiority that crushed my fragile spirit. A small crowd of onlookers whispered and giggled as I hobbled to my feet and scampered off toward the bathroom to hide in shame as the bully's mother smacked him in the back of the head and scorned him further.

"Aah you twyin'a git thuthpended!?"

"I ain't even hit 'eem that hard, Maw! He just a crybaby!"

In the middle of their fierce back-and-forth, a third voice, soft and calming, cut them off and gently pulled me back into the physical world.

"Good evening, everyone. The ceremony is now closed."

Despite her soothing voice, my pounding heart refused to calm down. With neither the energy nor the coordination to sit up, I lay motionless on my back and struggled to control my rapid breathing as the heavy feet of my cohorts shuffled past me toward the exit. My racing emotions blinded me from seeing that the schoolyard bullying, though it only occurred once, contributed to my progressively misanthropic view of the world, fueled by a long string of unfortunate incidents different in nature but similar in effect: emotional or physical suffering at the hands of others.

My breathing gradually returned to normal, and I opened my eyes to see the last few jittery silhouettes of stiff-legged zombies in their clumsy march toward the exit. One of the zombies — an absentminded young man, perhaps unaware of his presence on planet Earth — failed to contain the unbearable brightness of his flashlight, shining it directly into my face. Painful white light flooded my eyes, forcing them closed as my dilated pupils recoiled. A sheet of white burned into my retinas and persisted even behind my closed eyelids as the perpetrator sauntered by. My vision slowly recuperated just enough and just in time to see the perpetrator's lethargic silhouette exiting the hut and neglecting to shut the screen door behind him.

My misanthropic tendencies that I had yet to understand incited an involuntary, smart-aleck remark that erupted in my mind.

"Yo, if we could get some mosquitoes up in here, that'd be dope."

The words rang out with such clarity that I froze in shameful fright, unsure if I had inadvertently muttered it out loud. I hid in the anonymity of dark silence, but within minutes a mosquito attack forced me out the door despite my questionable balance.

As I stumbled through the uneven jungle paths, I locked my eyes on the ground immediately in front of my feet, scanning for the jungle's numerous pitfalls, and scanning for jungle creatures that might frighten me off balance. In the top of my peripheral vision, the bouncing bright light of a headlamp approached from off in the distance. I attempted to formulate the thought "I am in no condition for human interaction right now", but instead managed to muster only the one-word thought, "No..."

I froze in place like a deer in headlights. Even if the jungle had provided a path to flee, my limited mobility precluded any hope of escape. I shielded my eyes with one hand as the overwhelming brightness approached, and a familiar voice boomed from the blinding light.

"Hey there! I thought that was you. How was your experience tonight?"

His feet came to a standstill in the dirt path and dashed my hopes of a quick, minimal exchange of pleasantries in passing. I summoned all my mental strength but failed to produce a coherent response, and instead mumbled an affirmative hum that trailed off to nowhere.

"Mmm..."

Perhaps still out of whack himself, he failed to recognize the painful brightness that his headlamp inflicted upon me. As I grimaced and shielded my dilated eyes, he launched into a babbling monologue of incoherent nonsense, rambling about cosmic spiritual jibber-jabber that would have confused me even in a sober state of mind. His Gatling gun mouth assailed me with meaningless words that bounced off my forehead in rapid-fire succession and further disoriented me. I stood wobbling in silence, trying to mind my manners while enduring his maelstrom of babbling until I realized that he didn't even stop to breathe.

With no other options, I butted in.

"I, uh..."

He paused to let me speak.

"Neeeed...a toilet."

Though I used it as an excuse, it was the truth.

"Hah! All right then. I'll see you tomorrow, buddy. Good night!"

I attempted to match his enthusiasm but again only mustered the same affirmative hum that trailed off to nowhere, supplemented with squinted eyes and a farewell nod.

My head spun as I trudged back to my hut, ascended the stairs, strewed my personal effects about the bed, and then shed all my clothing onto the floor. Escalating rectal pressure suddenly approached emergency levels, roaring with an ominous gurgle as I made a stumbling dash for the toilet. Before I even sat down, an uncontrollable soft mush leaked from my hind parts and just barely landed in the toilet. When I secured my balance upon the plastic throne and relaxed my trembling sphincter, it unleashed a motley rush of watery feces intermittently punctuated by exploding pockets of wretched gas.

A gastrointestinal orgasm of alleviation fluttered through my quivering body as my emphatic sighs of relief bordered on moaning. I took a moment to recuperate, then began the long, arduous, acrobatic ordeal of wiping myself in the dark with the inadequate illumination of my mobile phone.

With that mess out of the way, I proceeded toward the bed and gathered the supplies necessary to exorcise a different type of demon. I offered Mother Ayahuasca one last chance to object, but she remained silent, so I commenced the uncouth ceremony of using clumpy sunblock as a makeshift lubricant to ejaculate into a vomit pale.

Throughout my post-pubescent life, testosterone-fueled bad ideas routinely masqueraded as good ideas, sometimes even as great ideas. The longer I denied myself sexual release, the more appealing a bad idea would sound, whether it was the ill-advised pursuit of an unscrupulous woman, the employment of a questionable contraception method, or the misguided notion to "enhance" masturbation using Tiger Balm. But as a reliable antidote, orgasm always exposed the idiocy of any such bad idea, no matter how convincing the earlier charade. The fast-acting potency of orgasm reliably laid bare the raw, stinking terribleness of a previously stellar-sounding idea, not minutes or hours afterward upon contemplative reflection, but immediately and involuntarily, before the contractions of ejaculation even began to wane. The powerful and sobering release would toss me into a tizzy where I swirled in confusion, conflicted by the simultaneous thrill of orgasm and pangs of shameful remorse.

But as I lay in the darkness of my jungle hut, with the demon exorcised and a mess upon myself, having broken the sacred vow of Ayahuasca abstinence, my only regret was that I hadn't done it sooner. I stood by my decision, and I sighed from relief, knowing that for the remainder of the ceremonies, unwelcomed visions of psychedelic lechery would haunt me no more.

Second Day of Rest

The murky darkness of dreamless sleep thinned out as my waking consciousness faded in, accompanied by dehydration and a headache that felt foreign, as if artificially implanted in my skull. I licked my parched lips and opened my eyes, allowing in a mild dose of indirect sunlight, unbearably bright and inexplicably painful. My eyes clamped themselves shut as I twisted around to face away from the light, and my lower back groaned with the same stiff soreness that often signals the onset of influenza.

An itchy burning sensation tingled across my legs, and they shouted for attention from beneath a haphazard pile of half-discarded blankets. Mental and physical exhaustion crushed me as I deliberated between two equally unappealing choices: expend energy to investigate my itchy legs, or conserve energy and simply weather the storm. The itchiness intensified as my waking consciousness fully materialized, prompting me to swat off my blanket and curl my legs upward for inspection. Insect bites of various sizes peppered my calves and thighs, possibly from mosquitoes, possibly from spiders, possibly from exotic Amazonian insects. I knew that scratching would not alleviate the irritation and would in fact worsen it, but I scratched anyway, indeed worsening it.

I swiveled out of bed and reached to put on the same shirt and pants that I had worn the day before, and I realized that I had not changed my socks or underwear for the last five days. The idea of fresh socks and underwear sounded appealing for a moment, but then I thought about the physical energy required to walk across the room and dig them out of my backpack, and the mere thought exhausted me. I also conceded that my current filthiness mostly stemmed from skipping the floral baths, not from my clothes. So for the sixth day in a row, I put on the same socks and underwear, and then dragged my weary feet out the door toward the dining hall.

Breakfast tasted wonderful but failed to ease the exhaustion which plagued me into the afternoon, when everyone gathered for our second group meeting. As with last time, we formed a circle inside the ceremonial hut and shared our experiences one by one to an attentive audience of our fellow participants. Unlike the cloud of hesitance that loomed about our first meeting, a refreshing air of trust and intimacy permeated the room right from the start, enlivening the same people who only four days prior had been nervous fidgeting strangers sitting in awkward silence and mutually averting eye contact.

Fatigue prevented me from sitting up, so instead I lay on my stomach and propped up my lifeless torso using the stilts of my arms. I surveyed the room and noticed several other participants who likewise appeared to be devastated by physical fatigue, or by lack of sleep, or by both.

But within minutes my physical ailments paled in comparison to the heartbreak of hearing participants share their personal histories of profound grief and trauma. Nothing in the entirety of my life compared to their agonizing ordeals: enduring a childhood of ruthless abuse, battling against decades of debilitating physical pain, witnessing the murder of family members. Slow tears rolled down the faces of speakers and listeners alike as a sorrowful symphony of sniffles played in the background.

Some recounted fruitless years of attempted recovery through traditional means of psychotherapy and antidepressants. Some confessed that they had been tempted by suicide, and that Ayahuasca had been their last-ditch effort. Some wept uncontrollably, both from the difficulty of retelling their horrific traumas, and from the elation of making real progress — for the first time ever — toward coping and recovery. I struggled to fight back the welling tears in my eyes as my quivering throat strangled itself, and the experience reminded me how lucky I've been in life.

When my turn came, I debated whether I should even share at all. Though I knew it was not a pity contest, I couldn't shake the embarrassment of lacking anything that compared to the heartbreaking testimonies of my predecessors. But with all eyes on me, I vacuumed up a deep breath through my nostrils and decided to share what little I had to offer: my paltry personal progress of liberation from fear, and acceptance of mortality. Survivor's guilt racked me as I teetered on the brink of tears, and my thin raspy voice repeatedly cracked like that of a pubescent teenager.

At the conclusion of the meeting, everyone released a collective sigh of relief that seemed to energize the group with positivity and hope. The uplifting rejuvenation persisted in me like a warm intoxication after the meeting's conclusion, even as my resurfacing soreness and fatigue escorted me back to my hut. The warm intoxication persisted for the remainder of the afternoon as I lay in bed, conserving my limited energy. It persisted through the evening as I devoured my first dinner in three days. And it persisted as I snuggled into bed at night, reflecting on the profound healing potential of Ayahuasca, and Western civilization's unforgivable crime against humanity in outlawing such a beneficial tool.

The day's sharing session forced a complete reevaluation of my world view, as all my negative experiences in life now felt trivial. I finally started to recognize my pessimism and misanthropy, and the absurdity of each. After hearing so many stories of grief, I realized that everyone has been hurt in one way or another, and that often times people who inflict pain probably do so as a subconscious coping mechanism for dealing with their own pain. Though I couldn't condone their actions, I now at least understood them, and the resentment and bitterness that I had unknowingly harbored inside me melted away into sympathy and forgiveness. A newfound peace of mind slowly lulled me to sleep, despite my increasingly weary and aching body that foretold trouble in the days ahead.

Sixth Night with Ayahuasca

Two distinct lucid dreams replayed in my mind as I awoke, but severe fatigue and soreness distracted me from reconstructing the fragmented dream details into a coherent narrative. My stomach growled an ambiguous complaint, partially from hunger, partially in recollection of its tumultuous contents of the past few days. Though I wanted to go eat the breakfast that awaited me, I chose to endure my hunger rather than expend the energy to get out of bed, and I would have stayed there motionless until lunchtime if not for a compulsory urge to urinate.

After emptying my bladder, I convinced myself to trudge to the dining hall and eat breakfast. A moderate portion of gruel and fresh fruit helped alleviate some of my discomfort and motivated me to join our group as the shamans gave a guided tour of the jungle, explaining via translator the many uses of the Amazon's diverse plant life. For fear of being eaten alive — not by jaguars, but by mosquitoes — I donned my usual long-sleeved pajamas with socks and shoes, doused from head to toe with DEET-free insect repellent. The shamans wore their traditional tribal garments, short-sleeved, some of them barefoot, with no insect repellent.

All at once, as if signaled by a rifle blast commencing open season, swarms of mosquitoes attacked in droves, indifferent to my DEET-free repellent, which somehow seemed to be attracting mosquitoes. My foolish appearance did not concern me as I struggled to shoo away the hordes by flailing in a spastic dance of constant twisting and turning, walking in place, flapping like a chicken, and swatting my limbs behind my head, over my shoulders, behind my back, and at my face.

A fellow participant who shared my distaste for mosquitoes had brought with him a professional adventurer's mosquito net mask, which he secured to his face. From the neck up, the impenetrable stronghold of netting protected him like a beekeeper's suit, but from the neck down he wore a sleeveless shirt, shorts, and sandals. He soon realized his gross folly, then attempted to improvise plates of armor by frantically scavenging large jungle leaves and tying them to his limbs using thin vines. His haphazard armor of vegetation proved useless, and the ravenous hordes effortlessly penetrated the gaping cracks in his loose defenses.

The participant in front of me wore a loose t-shirt, and upon his shoulder a trifecta of enormous mosquitoes leeched the blood from his flesh — straight through the cloth of his shirt — filling their red bellies at an alarming rate. Their proximity to each other proved to be a fatal mistake, as all three met their gruesome end in one swift smack of his palm, which smashed their swollen bellies and smeared a thick streak of blood across his hand and shoulder.

My botanical intrigue held out for only a few minutes before the urge to flee compelled me. Perhaps due to my diligent spastic dancing, I managed to escape without a single bite, and I spent the remainder of the day secluded in the sanctuary of my hut's mosquito netting, venturing out only for lunch, and forgoing my floral bath yet again.

As night fell and the ceremony drew near, my dwindling physical energy allotted me barely enough strength to douse myself again with ineffective insect repellent and then speed walk to the ceremonial hut.

The evening's brew tasted even worse than the previous five ceremonies. In addition to the usual overwhelming bitterness, it also contained an unexpected grainy texture, like sand in my mouth. My body insisted that I spit it out, but I fought the urge and forced down all three gulps.

Before everyone had even received their dose, one of the first participants shattered the silence of the illuminated room with preliminary dry heaving and guttural wheezing, and I wondered if my no-vomit streak would come to an end tonight.

The last participant tiptoed back to his mat, then the staff extinguished the lanterns, and darkness overtook the room. After thirty minutes of dark silence, a tingling anxiety seeped outward from my chest and abdomen, expanding to my limbs as I closed my eyes and prepared for blast off.

Glowing snowflake patterns of neon pink and purple danced for me, defying gravity as they twirled and spun in place, refusing to fall. Behind the shifting snowflakes, silent flashes of golden lightning illuminated a dark backdrop of billowing clouds. The psychedelic kaleidoscope soothed me, but from origins unknown a sudden tempest of noise infiltrated my mind: disjointed and rambling conversations, unfamiliar voices yelling at each other, revving engines and the angry honking of rush-hour traffic, jackhammers and backhoes tearing up asphalt, warning beeps of oversized vehicles in reverse, and two massive walls of static, one in each ear, sandwiching the multilayered cacophony.

My mental focus bucked like a wild bronco, yanking the reins from my grip. My thoughts darted to and fro in an uncontrollable, unpredictable zigzag of random directions like the erratic flight of a deflating balloon.

My backside suddenly smashed against the ground as if I had plummeted from above. The tremendous force of impact silenced the chaos in my mind and ripped the kaleidoscope visions from my sight. Confusion and disorientation surged through me in a spasm, as if I had jolted awake from a nightmare. My eyes searched across an unfamiliar black sky splashed with clouds, and I realized that an unknown but considerable amount of time had passed, and that I had just awakened from a deep state of unconsciousness. The missing chunk of time left no traces in my memory, and I slipped back into the raging whirlpool of mental noise.

The frantic thoughts continued right where they left off, now accompanied by a bewildering montage of fragmented and disarrayed visuals: familiar faces morphing into unfamiliar ones, flashbacks of actual memories spliced with fabricated scenes, organic cityscapes merging with landscapes, a parade of crawling insects and prowling animals, none of which corresponded to the relentless cacophony.

The songs of the shamans faded in, their voices offering a lifeline as I drowned in confusion. I latched on, but the female shamans thrashed at my ears with piercing shrieks. Rather than calming my mental disarray, their painful howling compounded it, and I recoiled with a cringe, dreading the thought of enduring such torture for several hours.

Another violent force of impact suddenly smashed into my backside and startled me into the world of visions. My frantic lungs sucked in a frightened gasp, and I realized that another chunk of unknown time had vanished from memory. Darkness surrounded me as I stumbled over the words of my confused thoughts, muttering unintelligible questions to no one.

"Wh...where...what the... I? Who...what is 'I'?"

Most of my memories had vanished, other than a vague recollection of my physical body and of traveling to Peru. I forfeited my attempts at coherent thought and tried to relax, but within seconds an unfamiliar scene faded in like a macabre, cinematic production.

My worm's-eye view peered up at a large clawfoot bathtub standing alone upon the weathered tiles of a dreary bathroom floor caked with mildew. Overhead, only one dim, flickering light bulb still clung to life, its waning glow further crippled by a thick layer of burnt yellow grime that coated the bulb. Neglected for years like the filthy tile floor, the light bulb struggled on its deathbed, only hours away from expiring like its fallen comrades.

In a slow and dramatic ascent, my point of view rose to reveal the contents of the bathtub: a mound of ice cubes protruding above the rim, and a naked young woman's pale body buried neck deep in a frigid bath of blood-red ice water. The weight of her head bent her limp neck into an awkward angle that cocked her head to the left. Cold sweat matted large and disheveled clumps of frizzled brown hair to her face like strands of stringy seaweed, between which her blue lips involuntarily mouthed something inaudible, and her closed eyelids twitched with the last glimmers of life. Her right hand rested upon the bathtub's filthy porcelain edge, and her slender fingers still clutched a bloodstained strip of crudely cut, crisscrossed metal grating. Loose shreds of her lacerated flesh dangled from the jagged rusty edges, and at the bottom corner a lone drop of coagulated blood — the last remnant of a once-flowing stream — appeared suspended in deliberation of whether to jump. Her left hand, sunken beneath the surface, rested upon the soft pillow of her upper thigh as life drained from the shredded flesh of her wrist, flooding the icy bath with deep crimson.

A frantic man crashed into the bathroom, slamming the wooden door against the sink, and his eyes bulged in horror as he lunged at her limp body.

"No, no! What have you done! WHAT HAVE YOU DONE!"

He clamped his quivering hands onto her face, straightened her neck, and then shook her head in desperation.

"WHAT HAVE YOU DONE!"

Her spasming eyelids fell closed as her pale, blue lips slurred a mumbling whisper.

"Mmmm...I...feeeel...so...coooold..."

He squeezed her frigid body with both arms, staining himself with crimson ice water.

"OH GOD, WHAT HAVE YOU DONE!"

He howled with remorse and trembled from hysteria as he yanked her limp body from the bath, spilling an avalanche of bloody ice water onto the grimy tile floor.

A wheezing death cry of gurgling pulled me back into the physical world, and the shrieking banshee cries of the female shamans lashed at my ears. A crippling abdominal pain wrenched my innards as an apocalyptic fit of diarrhea bludgeoned my sphincter, demanding every bit of my strength to contain the onslaught. I arched my back and grit my teeth in a self-paralyzing spasm of full-body clenching that exhausted me in mere seconds. As I collapsed onto my back, beads of sweat rolled down my forehead, and I spent the last of my strength swatting at them, convinced that they were mosquitoes.

Despair consumed me, and my subconscious groaned a plea for mercy that echoed with infinite reverb.

"Uuungh...maaake it stop...(-k't stop)...(-k't stop)...(-k't stop)..."

A distant and fragmented response in my own voice echoed back to me as if it had traveled backwards through time to reach me.

"...-er, -er, -er, -ender, -ender, -ender, surrender, -ender, -ender, -ender, -er, -er, -er..."

In a flash of mental clarity, I remembered that giving in was the only way out, and in the instant that I accepted my woes, they ceased to torment me. The painful intestinal cramping, the floundering off-key shrills, and the imaginary mosquito attacks all persisted unabated, but I transformed my perception of them from unbearable to inconsequential.

My physical body and the external world no longer concerned me, and they faded away as I drifted back into the world of visions.

At the top of a lush, grassy hill, a young tree stood alone in front of the sky's canvas of soft white and baby blue. Vibrant yellow dandelions speckled the surrounding green grass while monarch butterflies fluttered about, their magnificent orange hues glowing in the golden sunlight. Birdsong filled the air, and the picturesque scenery offered the perfect setting for a delightful afternoon picnic.

Under the tree's umbrella of shade, a gloomy woman sat perched like a gargoyle, with her knees to her chest, holding her face in her hands and arching her back as if ducking for cover. Her body trembled as a dark aura of ominous melancholy wafted in the air like the toxic fumes of smoldering plastic — a demonic silhouette that clashed against Mother Nature's idyllic backdrop.

Her identity eluded me as I approached with cautious steps and climbed toward the hilltop. The soft blades of grass bent and folded beneath my feet as I drew nearer without a word. I tried to announce my approach with a forced and conspicuous cough, but it failed to solicit her attention. She sat motionless except for her uncontrollable trembling, still holding her face in her hands, still fuming with an aura of darkness. The dandelions in her perimeter wilted and drooped as their brilliant yellow faded to moldy brown. In her shadow, swaths of green grass shriveled and retreated into the earth as if fleeing in terror from her noxious negativity, leaving a barren patch of parched soil at her feet.

I arrived within arm's length, hoping that she would turn to greet me or at least acknowledge my presence. A long moment of silence passed without even the sound of her visible whimpering, so I extended my arm, placing a gentle and comforting hand upon her shoulder.

She whipped her head around with a ferocious hiss and flashed two thin, finger-length fangs dripping with venom, like an agitated serpent about to strike. From the sides of her neck, an enormous cobra's hood of scaly flesh parachuted out and encompassed her snarling face. Fiery gold irises surrounded her thin vertical slits of jet-black pupils. Her sharp and piercing serpentine eyes tore into me, and I recognized them as my ex-girlfriend's. I immediately understood that I had done this to her, that she had mutated into a heinous monster because of the way I had treated her.

A tidal wave of guilt smashed into my face and chest, knocking the wind from my lungs, smothering me as I wheezed and gasped for air. My heart winced from excruciating regret as I acknowledged that I had caused her suffering: the anguish of heartbreak, the loneliness of abandonment, the disappointment of forlorn hope, and the lashing defense mechanism of distrust. Tears streamed down my face, and my lungs convulsed, desperate for air as I reached out with both arms to embrace her.

She hissed and writhed and struggled against me as I pulled her in close. She snapped her fangs at me as warning strikes that nearly pierced my neck, and I braced myself for the sting of her fangs sinking into my flesh, for the searing burn of her venom flooding my veins, for the crushing chest pains of my clotted blood stopping my heart. I acknowledged that I deserved it, as retribution for my crimes of unforgivable selfishness, for the devastating emotional damage and unbearable grief that I had inflicted upon her.

But as I wrapped my arms around her and pressed her chest against mine, her lethal fangs retracted, her fierce trembling and squirming gave way to a soft, whimpering sob, and she transformed into her benevolent human self. Her body heaved in my arms as we wept in silence, and though she twice attempted to, she couldn't bring herself to put her arms around me. I stroked the back of her head, pressing her cold face against the warmth of mine, and our streaming tears converged where our cheeks met.

Upon the cheeks of my physical body, the light caress of rolling teardrops pulled me out of the vision. My warped sense of hearing detected that somewhere nearby, perhaps in front of my own mat, a shaman sang as I wiped the tears from my face. With neither the physical strength nor the willpower to sit up, I lay on my back and toiled over whether I could ever make it up to my ex.

Time left me behind, but Ayahuasca intoxication did not, and a new, unrelated vision blindsided me like a freight train.

My stomach sank, and my eyes shot open to find myself face-to-face with the same type of stereotypical alien creature from a previous vision. His glossy black pair of softball-sized eyes reflected my distorted image back at me, and though he spoke not a word, he exuded a silent aura of extreme intelligence, like the palpable confidence and mastery oozing from a virtuoso on stage.

I broke the silence with a telepathic inquiry, directly from my consciousness to his.

"Are we able to communicate?"

His unflinching stare pierced into me, and his indecipherable expression bordered on grumpy. My intuition gleaned that he had received my message, but that his

171

conversational skills had atrophied as a result of eons of minimalistic, robotic communication with his fellow crotchety brethren, and that just like his punch-hole nostrils and tiny mouth-slit, his mental capacity for conversation had dwindled to a vestigial feature that served only to remind of his evolutionary past.

I sensed that likewise a lifetime of emotionally bankrupt interactions had atrophied his once-voracious appetite for intimacy and love. Sympathy took hold of me, and though nothing about his physical appearance struck me as cute or cuddly, I couldn't fight an irresistible urge to hug him out of love for my fellow living creature. I opened my arms and extended them outward while stepping forward to close the small gap between us. He neither welcomed nor resisted my approach, unflinching in his emotionless demeanor as I flung my arms around his oversized head and squeezed with an enthusiastic bear hug. His forehead pressed against my chest, and the warmth of my torso resuscitated his cold, corpse-like skin. Pulses of electrifying energy surged between us, out from my chest and in through his gigantic forehead, fueling his emotionally deficient body with long-lost vigor. I licked my lips and planted a wet, exaggerated kiss on the gray plateau of skin covering his dome, and after sucking a tight vacuum of air with my lips, I peeled off with a hearty and audible pop, accentuated by my emphatic vocalization.

"Mmmmmmwah!"

He squinted his enormous eyes and giggled like a toddler, unable to contain himself. The slit of his mouth curved upward into an adorable miniature smile, which he tried to hide behind his long thin fingers. We laughed together, giddy with uncontainable joy as I rocked us back and forth, and he wriggled in a playful, feigned attempt to squirm his massive head free from the grip of my bear hug.

The vision collapsed under the crushing sound of frantic heaving from across the room as some poor participant's convulsing body struggled to evacuate his stomach. After six or seven strenuous attempts that ousted only a light dribble of stomach acid, my exhausted cohort moaned with a quivering gasp of relief as his body finally conceded.

I slipped back into the world of visions to find that my alien friend had disappeared, and that my consciousness had detached from my body. I saw myself standing alone off in the distance on an elevated platform shaped like a serving platter: a flat oval surface supported by a thin beam shaped like an hourglass, which extended out of sight below. The isolated island platform stood several stories above ground level, with no connecting staircase or bridge or hint about how I had gotten there, forcing my assumption that I had been airlifted or teleported.

The platform comprised the center stage of a towering oval silo. Finely detailed trimmings and elaborate carvings decorated exquisite, bejeweled banisters and rows of seating that lined the walls, encircling me from a distance and stretching dozens of stories high and out of sight. The grandeur of the architecture and interior design rivaled that of Europe's most magnificent cathedrals, yet the presence of the stage and seats fueled my suspicion that I stood in some sort of theater.

I watched myself gazing out onto the surrounding rows, surveying my audience — a full house, every seat occupied by a large-headed creature like my giggly alien friend. Though I couldn't differentiate him from the thousands of others in attendance, I felt his presence and instinctively knew that he, as a senior official in his extraterrestrial homeland, had organized this performance for me to likewise resurrect the long-lost emotional capacity of his fellow brethren, just as I had for him.

173

My viewpoint hurtled through the air toward myself and snapped back into first-person perspective behind my eyes. The immense physical distance between me and my audience exacerbated the emotional distance between us, and countless rows of stern black eyes stared at me from afar, jabbing at me with impatient skepticism. The sea of spiritless faces clued me in that, just as the dawn of agriculture had negated the city dweller's need to hunt, these aliens too had evolved beyond a need for emotion, leaving it millennia behind; and, in the same way that a tribesman can teach a city dweller how to hunt, these aliens needed a creature like myself — someone still in touch with his primitive nature — to teach them how to laugh, through the lost art of comedy.

With no previous comedy experience, no prepared material, and no choice but to freestyle, I simply relinquished control to my subconscious, and a smooth stream of autopilot improvisation spilled forth. The words emerged inaudible, but in a visible current of illuminated glyphs that flowed from my mouth and spiraled upward through the oval interior as complete silence stifled the auditorium. I delivered the nonchalant setup to my first bit, and before delivering the punch line, I paused for suspense, mirroring the cold robotic demeanor of my bobblehead audience as I rotated around to face them all.

I could neither hear my own words nor read them as they materialized out of my mouth, but my first punch line launched the audience into an eruption of guffaws and a wave of shoulder heaving and knee slapping. The auditorium trembled from an earthquake of riotous hooting and hollering, bellowing laughter, and thunderous applause, and I, without pausing to let them catch their breath, continued with my nonchalant, autopilot monologue, not even sure if I was speaking English or Japanese.

My viewpoint zoomed out from the top of my head and sailed toward the unknown heights of the auditorium. I soared past row upon row of sold-out seating as the alien audience doubled over with laughter, ecstatic to be reunited with such a long-lost emotion. From my bird's eye view, the tiny speck of my physical body disappeared, and the surrounding theater seating faded to black.

My consciousness and physical body reunited, but something felt awry, as if waking from a coma, with a large chunk of recent memory erased. The shamans had concluded their songs, and my comedy performance felt like hours ago. A staff member announced the close of the ceremony, and several participants navigated their way out the door as I remained on my back, physically and mentally discombobulated, mulling over the contents of my heavily redacted memories.

My neighbor to the right adjusted his sitting position upon his mat, and my heightened sense of hearing amplified the soft rustling of his clothes. The sound tore into my ears, rattling me like a loudspeaker pressed against my head. At the same time, a shaman in the center of the room stood up, sending a small shockwave through the loose floorboard that ran beneath my lifeless body. The unexpected vibration in the floorboard, combined with the raucous sound of rustling to my right, duped me into thinking that my intoxicated neighbor must be wriggling toward my mat to cuddle with me.

Vibrating gradients of black obscured my vision and allowed my imagination to run wild. I envisioned my encroaching neighbor wriggling closer, and I attempted to shoo him away with gentle kicks, none of which connected. I withdrew my right leg and extended my right arm, shaking it all about in his direction, but my hokey-pokey dance only shooed away my own vomit pail, which skid across the wooden floorboards. The ruckus jolted me into focus and prompted the realization that I had only imagined the intruder, and that I should retreat to my hut before I embarrass myself further.

A sudden and frightening pressure of impending explosive diarrhea confirmed that I needed to retreat to my hut immediately. Panic temporarily overcame my Ayahuasca intoxication and aided me in my wobbly scurry through the jungle. Surging adrenaline blurred away the details, and suddenly I found myself in the bathroom of my hut, struggling to yank down my long pajama pants without falling over, and without leaking from between my buttocks. The primal fear of soiling myself empowered me to clamp shut my quivering sphincter until I crashed onto the plastic toilet seat, nearly snapping it off the loose hinges as a seemingly endless deluge of filth blasted forth from my rear.

I lost track of time as I wiped and wiped, and after a quarter roll of toilet paper, my chafed anus begged me to stop. I obliged despite a looming suspicion that my last wipe wasn't white, and that suspicion soon proved moot when a renegade squirt of diarrhea slipped through my defenses and seeped into my underwear. I lurched back to the toilet, discarded the soiled undies into the trash, wiped my chafed anus yet again, and then put on a clean pair of underwear for the first time in a week.

Soreness and exhaustion engulfed me as I crawled into bed, but my racing mind prohibited sleep, so I cued up a relaxing playlist of solo piano, and then fumbled my headphones into a crooked arrangement upon my head. The melody's intro of usually soft and soothing notes lashed at my ears with jarring high-voltage jolts, and my disarrayed senses twisted the beautiful composition into auditory torture — a sour disharmony like the clashing notes of a piano out of tune. I tried switching to a different pianist, but that too sickened me, forcing me to give up on solo piano.

I switched genres and cued up a progressive rock album, knowing that it wouldn't serve as a lullaby, but curious if it would sound as heinous as piano. Though I had heard the album hundreds of times before, the explosive opening chord startled me with stunning freshness and novelty, as if I had been deaf my entire life and were hearing music for the first time. The song as a whole, as well as each individual instrument, sounded utterly new, and a constant stream of fantastic audio surprises raced past me like whizzing spaceships, faster than I could comprehend.

My subconscious fastened an individual thread of attention to each piece of the song: the lead, backup, and bass guitars; the hi-hat, crash cymbal, ride cymbal, snare, bass drum, hanging toms, and floor toms; the melodies and arpeggios of the piano and synthesizer; the lead, backup, and harmonic vocals. My subconscious deconstructed the song into these individual components, and I saw them — each thread of attention — as a vibrating and illuminated audio wave. The fluid, dancing threads of light comprised a visual mixing console as an audio engineer would see, and my mind tracked the vibrations of each thread individually, as well as their marvelous symbiotic relationships with each other. An unfamiliar tingling buzz of excitement and suspense surged through me as the song's tension peaked, the vibrating threads of light magnified into explosive lightning bolts, and the climactic crescendo tore into me with pulsating electric warmth that fluttered in my chest and took my breath away. The beauty of the ensemble and its majestic synergy — orders of magnitude greater than the sum of its parts — dazzled me to the point of paralysis as the cornucopia of audio euphoria poured into my ears.

Each song thereafter launched me into an equally epic audiovisual journey, each phenomenal in its own unique way. I relished in what felt like audio orgasms through the first two-thirds of the album, but then insurmountable fatigue and a tyrannical fit of yawning implored me to sleep, appropriately timed with the conclusion of track number nine, titled "Blackout". My lethargic hand nudged the headphones off my head, and within minutes I drifted into a serene and dreamless void of consciousness, blissfully unaware of the misery that awaited me in the morning.

Seventh Night with Ayahuasca

My achy bones and sore muscles groaned, smothered by their own unbearable weight, begging me to lie still. I refused to open my eyes, holding out hope that my physical agony merely stemmed from the residual pain of a profoundly uncomfortable dream.

A thunderstorm of gas erupted in my lower abdomen as it trampled the decimated corridors of my digestive tract. Smaller gas clouds consolidated into a mega cloud that stubbornly loitered at the sharp turns in my intestines and demanded that I help facilitate its passing. The intestinal discomfort momentarily exceeded my musculoskeletal discomfort, and I forced my creaky body to roll over like a decrepit old dog long weary of doing tricks.

My pelvis and lower spine wallowed in misery as I twisted my hips. A flulike soreness ravaged every moving muscle and conjoining skeletal structure, resonating outward with a ripple of discomfort that lingered long after I stopped moving. I dreaded the inevitable task of rising from bed, and I lay motionless in procrastination, already exhausted.

The unclogged mega cloud of gas blurted out an obscene grumble as it rounded the corner of my intestines and lurched onward, quickly filling my rectum, where it mingled and conspired with a slushy mess of free-floating debris.

I hoisted myself into a sitting position, and a new brigade of discomfort bludgeoned my organs from the inside. At the same time, dizzying lightheadedness and a pounding headache momentarily distracted me from the impending need to evacuate my bowels, until another wicked rectal grumbling compelled me to the toilet.

What my bowel movement lacked in volume it made up for in ferocity, blasting out with the erratic explosiveness of a repeatedly misfiring rifle. I waited in silent helplessness until my sphincter spasms subsided, and a prolonged eerie silence suggested that the storm had passed. But when I reached for the roll of toilet paper, another violent rectal misfire startled my hand away from the roll, back to its timid resting position upon my knee.

After fully evacuating my bowels, my body afforded me only enough energy to lurch back to bed, and even my lethargic strides took a toll on me. With no appetite to motivate me and no energy to propel me along the impossible odyssey to the dining hall, I scoffed at the idea of breakfast and collapsed back into bed. Lying motionless and concentrating on nothingness provided some solace for an hour or so, but then another riot erupted inside my rectum, with the same alarming urgency as before. My body ached at the thought of physical movement, but I once again trekked the miserable journey back to the toilet, only because it required less energy than constantly clenching my chafed anus.

Arduous journeys to the toilet at one-hour intervals became the norm. Squirt by squirt, the mushy mountain of diarrhea and toilet paper and sawdust grew so tall that I feared filling up the toilet bucket, forcing me to forego the sawdust and simply let each new round fester on top of the previous. This process repeated throughout the day, and I ventured out of my hut only once, for a piddling portion of lunch, which I force-fed myself, and which sustained my relentless flow of diarrhea until sundown.

The ceremony drew near, and I buried my day's worth of excrement in sawdust, careful to leave enough room for a post-ceremony calamity.

Though the flowing river of diarrhea had slowed to a trickle, an onslaught of internal discomfort, musculoskeletal aches, digestive cramps, and crippling fatigue perpetuated my miserable condition. My body cried out in agony as I dragged myself toward the ceremonial hut. My weary leg muscles lacked the strength to tread lightly, dumping each foot down with a forlorn and graceless thump that pummeled the whole of my skeleton, and the repeated impacts jarred me like recurring head-on collisions.

Along the way, I toiled over the serious dilemma at hand: despite my considerable investments in time and money and effort to be here, I dreaded the thought of drinking Ayahuasca in my current condition. I reflected on the taxing journey by plane, bus, boat, and then by foot just to arrive in the jungle, the thousands of US dollars in airfare and retreat cost, the rarity of the opportunity, and the potential for profound introspection. But all those reasons failed to mitigate the cruel punishment of sentencing myself to four hours of writhing on that hard, wooden floor as Ayahuasca tore through my enfeebled body and wrenched my aching guts. I gagged at the mere thought of smelling Ayahuasca, and I spared myself the unfathomable thought of drinking it, conceding that, much to my chagrin, I would have to sit on the sidelines for this ceremony.

The staff, however, wouldn't stand for it. Plead as I might, they insisted in a hushed but stern voice that I should at least drink half a dose, stressing that I would regret the squandered opportunity, and asserting that Ayahuasca would heal my ailments — a claim that struck me as absurd. But knowing very little of Western medicine, and even less of Amazonian shamanism, I caved in and agreed to half a dose, with an oppressive cloud of reluctance hanging overhead.

In an effort to alleviate my symptoms, the head shaman blew a blessing of tobacco smoke onto my tiny dose for the evening, and I swallowed the stinging brew with surprising ease, perhaps because thus far I had been downing quadruple the amount.

181

Several pairs of curious and confused eyes watched me return the suspiciously tiny cup and shuffle back to my mat. Immediately upon returning, my muscles gave up, and I collapsed into the least uncomfortable position that I could find: lying on my back, legs extended outward, knees slightly bent, hands folded across my abdomen. I distracted myself from my pervasive soreness by focusing on the black emptiness behind my closed eyes, and I hoped for a hasty onset of visions.

An unknown amount of time passed before I suddenly found myself sitting alone on an invisible bench, surrounded by cold and empty darkness. A cool tingle ran down the back of my neck, tightening my skin into goose bumps and standing my hair on end. I held my gaze straight ahead, afraid to immediately look to my right side, from whence I felt the overbearing presence of something sitting next to me in silence.

My subconscious reassured me with a whisper.

"Whatever it is, it can't hurt you."

With a slow swivel to the right, I turned to face the bulging, basketball-sized shoulder of a tremendous ogre man sitting beside me, motionless. Coarse bristles of wiry hair covered his rough and weathered Caucasian skin, and his intimidating enormity fully eclipsed me. His powerful forearms, thicker than my thighs, seemed to swell with his every breath, as did the mountain of trapezius muscle that jutted upward from his shoulders and buried his neck.

His gradually sloping forehead formed a gorilla brow that extended over his eye sockets like a thick canopy, hiding beneath it a pair of sunken eyes. His immense jaw widened his head into a pear shape, from the top of which protruded a single bushel of hair like a carrot sprout. He exacerbated his doofus appearance with a blank, absentminded stare, but what he appeared to lack in intelligence he more than compensated for in power. His refrigerator-sized torso of solid muscle pulsated with strength, and his monstrous hands dwarfed my head, which he could have crushed between his fingers.

He slowly turned to face me, and his neck muscles creaked like a massive chamber door drawing open for the first time in centuries. The crevice between his protruding brow and his prominent cheek bones afforded us only a narrow slit through which to make eye contact, and his sunken eyes hid in the shadows of his skull.

He seemed indifferent to my presence, allowing me a moment to ponder how to greet him.

"Well, he's a huge, weird-looking dude...who probably represents something. So...let's start there."

He held steady his apathetic, unflinching stare as I cleared my throat and opened my mouth to speak.

"What do you represent?"

His jaw barely moved, as if rusted stiff, and he parted his lips only wide enough for muffled syllables to dribble out like slow-rolling drool.

"Nuh-thin'. I'm just a huge, weird-lookin' dude."

He punctuated the statement with several seconds of stern, unblinking eye contact before turning his creaky neck and his empty gaze back toward the blackness in front of us. The finality of his statement, and the implication that he had read my mind, convinced me to likewise turn my gaze back toward the blackness in front of us. I stared off into nothingness and contemplated if the brief encounter contained any hidden meaning, but then a sudden itchiness flared up in my ear canal.

Unlike previous ceremonies, the evening's tiny dose of Ayahuasca had left my basic motor skills intact, and I raised a nimble hand to the side of my head. My index finger traced the contour of my ear and then attempted to scratch the inside, but an unexpected blockade obstructed my ear canal, which had swollen shut at some point during the day, unbeknownst to me. I prodded and scraped at the hard lump of swollen flesh but failed to satiate the itch within, and then suddenly, as if falling through a trap door, I crashed back into the world of visions.

Ayahuasca thrust me into a forgotten memory from early childhood, and as a toddler I stood next to our family's station wagon on the side of a busy street as speeding cars whizzed past, each zooming whoosh startling me over and over. My mother stood beside me and focused her worried gaze across the roof of the station wagon, and I focused my attention on her as she furrowed her brow, folded her arms, and shook her head back and forth. My youthful naivete precluded me from understanding the situation, but my mother's shaky voice and restless fidgeting fueled my burgeoning distress.

A police officer stood across from us, jotting down notes as my mother grappled with her words and thoughts.

"I don't know. I don't know what it was. It must've, some...something must've hit the windshield."

I clasped my tiny hands onto my mother's pant leg, and a crushing fear suffocated my fragile little body. Helplessness and confusion swirled inside me as I struggled to fight back an imminent eruption of tears.

The scene abruptly shifted, and I found my same toddler self thrust into a different forgotten childhood memory, standing at thigh height next to my mother on a middle-school playground. Tears streamed down my cheeks, and I clutched onto my mother's leg, wailing as I looked up at the coalescing beard of blood that poured from her nostrils, down her face, and down the front of her neck. The unfamiliar, bloody face of my own mother horrified me, and I hid my face in the side of her leg as herds of schoolchildren screamed and shrieked, running past us like gazelles fleeing from a lion. The relentless snarling and barking of a ferocious dog further fueled the pandemonium, and I tightened my tiny clutches around my mother's leg as someone behind me shouted in a trembling voice of concern.

"Oh my God! Ma'am, are you okay!?"

The roaring pandemonium exploded with a pop like a balloon touching flame, bursting into utter silence as the scene once again transformed into a different childhood memory, and I found my same toddler self — now smiling, happy, and carefree — skipping down the halls of my preschool. My gleeful footsteps faded in from the silence, squeaking against the cheap vinyl floor, and my egg salad sandwich bounced back and forth inside my plastic superhero lunch box. From the depths of my subconscious, a distant reverberation of my mother's voice echoed in my mind.

"Nicky, it's not going to heal if you keep licking it."

For days she had been trying to convince me to stop licking my moustache of chafed skin above my upper lip — a self-inflicted wound resulting from a mysterious compulsion to frequently swipe my tongue back and forth like windshield wipers across my upper lip.

My mother's warning still echoed in my mind as I stopped mid-trot in the hallway. I crossed my eyes to look down my nose at my extended tongue, which I bent upward, pressed against my glowing red moustache of chafed skin, and then wiped back and forth with all my strength. The saliva softened and reopened the cracked skin of my upper lip, and the heavy friction of my vigorous licking wiped away what miniscule layer of skin had healed. The cool, stinging air irritated my raw skin, but a confounding gratification anesthetized the pain.

The shrieking falsetto of a female shaman yanked me back into the physical world. Unbeknownst to me, she had parked herself in front of my mat, and her disharmonious assault of piercing notes, much like Ayahuasca itself, tasted unbearably bitter to my ears. Also like Ayahuasca, her shrieking song punched me in the gut with a heavy fist of nausea, and I winced on the brink of dry heaving. Initially I fought the urge to vomit, distracting myself with calm thoughts and deep breaths, but then I reminded myself that I must accept whatever comes, and that barfing up Ayahuasca can even feel therapeutic, according to my fellow participants.

I eased my defensive resistance, opened my mind, and gulped down the bitter melody as she poured it into my ears. Her cracking voice rattled my skull, but the more I relaxed, the more palatable her song became. The morbid bitterness of her voice receded to a more tolerable level comparable to the off-key floundering of drunken karaoke — a bitterness that I could swallow thanks to my years in Japan. Though her song initially felt excruciating and endless, she surprised me with a pleasant outro and an abrupt conclusion. She took a gentle hold of my head, blew a wet breath of scented water upon it and then between my outstretched hands. The last traces of my nausea vanished, and she shuffled over to my neighbor as I lay down and sunk into a new vision.

Soft and flowing curtains draped an ornate four-poster Victorian bed suited for royalty. The dark veil of night shrouded the bedroom with ominous blackness, and a thick fog of evil loomed in the frigid air. Upon the soft mattress and superfluous pillows of the extravagant bed, an unfamiliar young woman lay on her back, buried to her neck in thick blankets. Her unblinking eyes peered out from her paralyzed face, unable to scream. Dreadful fright seized her body and robbed her naturally pale skin of all its color, casting her flesh a ghastly white. Her rigid body, still warm with life but frozen with horror, lay motionless in the bed like a corpse in a casket.

The unbearable panic and confusion of her sleep paralysis surged through me as I watched helpless from afar and shivered from flashbacks of my own horrible bouts with sleep paralysis. I knew from experience that if only she could lift a finger to wake herself, she would snap out of it and end the living nightmare. But I also knew the impossibility of lifting a finger when trapped beneath that invisible, smothering blanket of abominable weight constricting her like a full-body straitjacket. She tried to squirm free but couldn't, unable to move anything other than her frantic eyes while drowning in the torturous dread of being mummified alive.

At the foot of the bed, a tall shadowy figure draped in a black cloak stood with his back to me, facing her with his arms perched above his head in a menacing attack pose. His long bony fingers arched downward at her, casting his hex of paralysis in preparation to pounce on her helpless body and ravage it to his wicked delight.

I slowly circled around to identify the woman's tormentor, and as I glided across the room in silence, the entire bedroom scene paused, suspended in animation like an immersive diorama, a three-dimensional slice of frozen space extracted from the reels of time.

At the head of the bed, I saw from the tormented woman's perspective the grisly incubus who towered over her. His shiny helmet of a head resembled the round shell of an enormous beetle and reflected the pale moonlight that crept into the room. A black ring of large and protruding spider eyes encircled the perimeter of his skull, and each of his countless eyes likewise reflected the faint moonlight, casting a nefarious twinkle of malevolent lecherous desire. A long and dense beard of thick black tentacles draped from his nose and cheeks, shrouding whatever ungodly orifice might lie beneath, while his slimy mess of tentacles wriggled and frothed with anticipation.

Someone from across the room launched into an exasperating attempt to vomit, drowning out the powerful voices of the singing shamans, and tearing me from my vision. He struggled through a dozen fruitless gurgling throat spasms until his whimpering body gave up and collapsed, and his hysterical heaving subsided into exhausted gasps for breath.

The world of visions faded back in, and my reflection stared back at me with droopy bloodshot eyes as I stood in front of my bathroom mirror, unconcerned with my sloppy job of brushing my teeth in preparation for bed. My ex-girlfriend stood to my right, also unconcerned with her own sloppy job of brushing her teeth. Our naked and sweaty bodies evidenced our indulgences of the evening, and my dehydration evidenced the excessive amount I had drunk, as she had requested at the start of the night.

"C'mon...I wanna see you really drunk! We've got plenty of wine, it's just the two of us, and you don't have to work tomorrow."

"Mmm, all right, if you insist...I'll make a spectacle of myself. But only for you. And no refunds!"

We both wobbled as we stared into our own reflections in the mirror, standing within a finger's length of each other, side by side in silent denial, neither of us wanting to acknowledge our impending and indefinite separation: my solo departure from the country. It loomed overhead like a black raincloud, stewing and waiting to unleash its relentless downpour of melancholy. At the time of the actual experience, I had hidden behind my emotional barrier, thus protecting me from the true gravity of the situation, but as I relived the experience in this Ayahuasca vision, stripped of my emotional barrier, just like her I stood defenseless against the inevitable deluge of sorrow.

I struggled to stifle an involuntary sigh of quivering heartache as I lowered my gaze and swapped my toothbrush into my other hand. I wrapped my arm around her waist, and I pulled her warm naked body next to mine. In the instant that the curvature of her soft hip pressed against the side of my thigh, our unspoken but profound mutual grief coursed between us like a frigid electrical current. We both looked up, straight ahead into each other's eyes in the mirror, and her innocent gaze pierced into me like an ice pick. I forced a goofy smile that parted the toothpaste bubbles on my lips, in hopes of distracting her from the tears welling in my eyes. I desperately fought back the emotions, knowing that if I broke down, she would too, and though I couldn't bear to hold it all in, I couldn't bear to hurt her any more than I already had.

Steadily flowing tears rolled down my cheeks from the corners of my closed eyes, and my fluttering chest heaved as I drew in deep breaths. One by one the shamans bowed out of their dissonant chorus, and I lost track of time as I mulled over the implausible notion of ever making it up to my ex. I knew that I couldn't undo the pain, but I also knew that I had to do something.

Though mild compared to previous nights, a diarrhea alarm forced me into an intense clench that wrung out the last few tears from my soggy eyes. I arched my back into a clumsy bridge pose that, despite ill form, aided in sealing off my sphincter valve. After a few seconds I relaxed my posture, surprised and delighted by the brevity of the maelstrom.

In the short span of a few minutes, the emotionally wrenching vision, the fading songs of the shamans, the waning psychoactive effects of my small dose, and the diarrhea alarm all combined into a perfect storm of sobriety — a stunning jolt of clarity that struck me without warning. Soft moonlight offered just enough illumination for my jitter-free eyes to trace the silhouettes of my neighbors, and from the center of the hut a calm whisper gently wedged into the silence of the room.

"Good evening, all you lovely people. The ceremony is now closed."

The dried river of tears upon my cheeks had left behind a thin layer of crusty tear flakes. As I brushed them from my face with two effortless strokes, I realized that unlike the conclusion of every other ceremony thus far, I had full use of my limbs. Sitting up, which had thus far been a laborious task, proved trivial and even refreshing. My balance held steady as I rocked forward into a low squat, scooped up my belongings, and rose to standing without even a wobble.

Muscle aches and full-body soreness still plagued me, but I strode with confident steps toward the exit, and unlike the shadowy silhouettes of my stumbling cohorts in front of me, I gracefully descended the staircase without the aid of the banister or a flashlight. At the base of the steps, I fished out my footwear from the mountain of sandals and then stepped aside to let the wobbly zombies fish for theirs. My balance and coordination astounded me as I slipped on my shoes one-handed while balancing on one leg — an unprecedented post-ceremony feat.

I set out along the dark jungle path for the seventh and final time, thrilled to find the formerly arduous journey now effortless — the once treacherous pitfalls now nothing more than minor bumps and ditches. A small chortle bubbled out of my throat like an unexpected belch as I envisioned how ridiculous I must have looked stumbling home after each of the previous six ceremonies, like a bumbling apelike forest jester entertaining all the creatures of the jungle.

In a flash, I saw the lizards and rodents and snakes and frogs, the bushes and shrubs, the porcupine tree, all keeling over with laughter as I stumbled past on previous nights. Two owls perched upon a tree branch spotted my stumbling silhouette of five nights ago, and one owl nudged the other with his wing, plotting to tease me.

"Aye yo, check this out. I'mma swoop overhead and scare the shit out this fool!"

I laughed to myself and conceded that indeed they had nearly scared the excrement out of me.

My nimble legs carried me back to my hut in record time, without incident. I disrobed, cast my clothes to the floor, and then strolled to the toilet with no fear of soiling myself. The plastic throne creaked as I sat upon it and awaited commencement, which took considerable time compared to previous nights.

The morbid stench of Ayahuasca diarrhea wafted into my nostrils and forced out of me a disgusted chuckle of repulsion. I cringed at not just the stench, but at my entire bodily foulness — head to toe — which resulted partly from the retreat's policies, and partly from my absentmindedness. Ten days without fingernail clippers or soap or toothpaste or tweezers had left me with black dirt packed beneath my barbaric fingernails, a sticky film of accumulated sweat and insect repellent coating my body, a residual layer of Ayahuasca grime upon my gums and teeth, and a wild, villainous unibrow.

Yet despite my abysmal personal hygiene, despite the flu-like affliction still ravaging my body, and despite the revolting filth trickling from my chafed and weary anus, euphoria overpowered everything. These ten grueling days had taught me more about myself than ten years of self-reflection. My mind throbbed with a newfound sense of self-awareness, a proud sense of accomplishment, and an extreme level of motivation, the likes of which I had seldom felt before, if ever.

The major turning points of my life replayed in my mind, and I mumbled to myself the realization that, all thanks to a hideously tasting magic potion, this had been the most profound and the most beneficial experience of my life. And in the same breath, I mumbled a serious assertion to myself that, unless administered via enema or nasogastric tube, I would never partake of Ayahuasca again.

Epilogue

During the first three months after returning from the jungle, I struggled to articulate a satisfactory answer to the most frequent question regarding my Ayahuasca experience: "So what did you get out of it?"

The limited tool of language seemed inadequate for the staggering task of expressing something so subjective, so otherworldly, and something that I myself didn't fully grasp. Furthermore, the fear of sounding like a lunatic worried me enough that initially I restrained myself to only two assertions: that it had been an extremely beneficial experience, and that, after forcing me to plow through four rolls of toilet paper in less than a week, Ayahuasca had renewed my appreciation for solid bowel movements.

But as I write this epilogue, the question of what I gained from the experience has been gestating in my mind for nine months, and like the soft head of a fetus nudging against my dilating mental cervix, the answers now feel fully developed and ready for delivery.

Before venturing to the Amazon, it had been roughly ten years since I last cried. Over that decade or so, despite heartbreaking relationships, the deaths of loved ones, and other misfortunes that warranted an emotional response, I never had to wipe away any tears, because the tears never came. I didn't know why, and I didn't give it much thought, aside from an absurd assumption that I had simply outgrown emotions. I didn't realize that my rusted and defective tear ducts were only the external symptom of a systemic problem: the entirety of my emotional plumbing had become calcified and clogged by hairy clumps of psychological resistance, and by moldy sludge of stubborn denial.

But much like industrial grade drain opener, in terms of effectiveness and perhaps even in terms of taste, Ayahuasca tore through me and annihilated my emotional blockages. During those seven nights, I cried more than I had in my entire adult life. And then I cried five more times while writing this book. I shed tears of elation, tears of sorrow, tears of liberation, and tears of regret, but all of them were meaningful tears, from which I learned something about myself, and from which I resolved to become a better person.

During the ceremonies, Ayahuasca obliterated my sense of self, stripped me of my biases and preconceived notions, and provided a lens of frightening realism, allowing me to not only see with lucid clarity my own actions from an outside perspective, but to also feel their devastating impact from the perspective of others. As a direct result I now find myself more aware of my words and actions, more careful with them, and more conscious of how they affect others.

In my mid-twenties, my ability to recall both short-term and long-term memories took a nosedive and steadily worsened year after year — an affliction that, despite occasional concern from friends, I casually wrote off as an unavoidable drawback of getting older. I assumed that my lost memories had forever vanished along with my declining cognitive abilities, but I see now that I never lost any memories. Rather, an oily layer of accumulated mental soot had coated the windowpane of recall through which I had been looking, and though all my memories were still intact behind the dirtied glass, I could no longer see them clearly.

But Ayahuasca annihilated the sticky blackened grime from my pane of recall and provided a sparkling clear window through which I can now see my once-estranged memories that stretch all the way back to early childhood.

Every few months a new memory spontaneously resurfaces, involving some boneheaded blunder or inconsiderate misdeed of mine from five, ten, even fifteen years ago. Some were minor discourtesies, like neglecting to say thank you, and some were egregious offenses, like leaving my friend stranded at the airport in a foreign country where he didn't speak the language. All these wrongdoings somehow sailed under my radar at the time, as I pranced about in my bubble of oblivious egocentrism. However, I have since reached out and apologized to those I had wronged, some of whom had trouble remembering the offense because so much time had passed.

After tracing my emotional footprints of the past, I now see that my former fear of intimacy stemmed from having my own heart broken, a subject curiously absent from my Ayahuasca visions. I realized that the resulting defense mechanism, which was supposed to protect me, was instead prohibiting me from living a more fulfilled life, and I now find it much easier to open up emotionally, especially with those from whom I had needlessly distanced myself.

I realized that for my entire adult life, I had been subconsciously insulating myself from the thought of death, both my own and that of loved ones. But Ayahuasca forced me to confront death head-on by experiencing it firsthand, in a simulation so convincing that it eliminated my fear of death, because now I feel like I already died once, and it fascinated me more than it scared me. And though I know it will still be difficult to handle the deaths of loved ones, I feel significantly more prepared for their inevitable deaths, which I now acknowledge and accept.

The theme of loose bowels ran throughout my seven nights with Ayahuasca, and I came to see parallels between that and mortality. I now think of life as a coast-to-coast car ride through vast, open countryside, and I view the inevitable deaths of loved ones as an incurable affliction of occasional but morbid diarrhea. Every so often during the car ride, I pass a rest stop where I have two choices: acknowledge the affliction by pulling over and relieving the unpleasant pressure, or suppress it and just keep driving, frightened by the potential horrors of a public bathroom: the sticky layer of fresh urine and putrefied bodily fluids covering the floor and peeling off onto the heels of patrons; the pungent casserole of excrement that coats the toilet seat and basin; the only available roll of toilet paper sopping on the floor, soaked in a puddle of unidentifiable orange-brown goo.

The terrifying thought of such a filthy facility had deluded me into thinking that I didn't have diarrhea, and so for the first thirty percent of my cross-country drive, I bottled up the pressure, pretended like it didn't exist, sped past each rest stop, and constantly fought back the urge to wince from the accumulated pressure swelling within me. But after drinking Ayahuasca — after being forced into the rest stop's bathroom — I found that it wasn't the dreadful cesspool that I had imagined, and that addressing my runny bowels liberated me from my self-inflicted misery. I see now that the pain of suppressing the problem had already eclipsed the unpleasantness of simply dealing with it, and that I also ran the risk of devastation by an uncontainable fit of catastrophic diarrhea that could have ruined my entire journey.

During my first five nights with Ayahuasca, I learned that the combination of repressed sexual instincts and a potent psychedelic can spawn bewildering and salacious scenes incomparable to anything I had previously experienced or imagined. I learned that if I'm going to take a psychedelic for introspective purposes, I should rub one out beforehand.

Despite my best online research efforts, I never found a conclusive answer as to whether cats produce endogenous DMT.

Ayahuasca didn't cure my flu-like ailments on the seventh ceremony, nor did it cure my recurring neck and shoulder problem. Ayahuasca also didn't squelch my dislike for mosquitoes, but it did empower me with the strength to accept that which I cannot change. Certain sounds, such as crying babies and screaming children, open-mouth chewing and any sort of slurping, used to irritate me to the brink of aneurysm, but now I find the formerly torturous sounds to be more tolerable, and sometimes even laughable. Rather than resisting them, I can now sometimes embrace them, which was previously unfathomable.

Likewise, the experience empowered me with the strength to let go. I now find myself unfazed by, and eager to move on from, things that used to frustrate me: poor customer service, broken promises, arguments, inconsiderate or absentminded road etiquette, and so forth. I realize now that latching on to those things only prolongs their negative effects, and that I can instantly thwart that negativity by letting go and moving on. In understanding my former misanthropy, I now see that many of the alleged offenses amounted to nothing more than honest mistakes, the kind that I myself probably make on a regular basis.

Ayahuasca instilled in me a love of plant life, and the mere presence of plants now fills me with subtle heartwarming affection, like the good company of family and friends. Five months after returning home from the Amazon, I surprised myself by climbing a tree for the first time in my adult life, and as I sat perched like a leisurely monkey, entirely sober, with my bare feet dangling and my palms resting upon the thick branch, I felt the rough bark not as the dead wooden surface of an inanimate object, but as the living, multiplying cells of a biological organism just like myself. The soft rustling of leaves in the wind and the gentle creaking of the sturdy tree limb pacified me like a cat's purr, and my hair stood on end, electrified by a startling affinity that I had thought only possible with my fellow mammals. Though I don't often find myself climbing trees, my newfound affinity for vegetation has enhanced my daily enjoyment of life, whether I am driving alongside a lush green forest, or simply staring at a lone tree outside my kitchen window.

Ayahuasca destroyed my desire for alcohol, but not my enjoyment of it. I still drink socially, and I still enjoy it, but the once-common thought "I want a drink" has disappeared without a trace, along with my once-common inclination to overindulge. Ayahuasca provided an inward journey of introspection and a profound expansion of consciousness, whereas heavy alcohol consumption now strikes me as an outward escape away from myself and as a profound retardation of consciousness.

I realized that throughout my relationship with my ex, I had cowered behind the stone wall of my emotional barrier. She had opened her heart to me, but my fear of intimacy never allowed me to open up to her, causing a massive imbalance in our relationship, and fooling me into believing the absurd idea that the breakup wouldn't be so bad. I can never undo the pain that I caused her, but after I returned home from the jungle, I flew her out to Hawaii so that I could offer my sincere apology face to face, and she somehow found the strength to forgive me.

Lastly, I had to retract my assertion from nine months ago where I swore that if I ever tried Ayahuasca again, it would have to be via enema or nasogastric tube. The long-term benefits of this journey have been so profound that, even if it means suffering through that awful taste again, I look forward to seven more nights with Ayahuasca.

About the Author

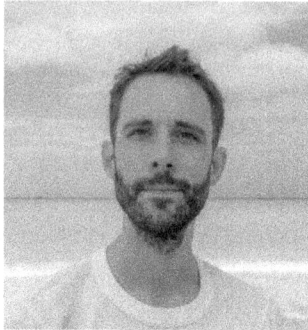

Nicholas Floyd was born in the Midwest of the United States of America, where he lived an uneventful two decades until, as a young college student, he received sage advice from a fellow Midwestern native who had fled to California and who insisted that Nicholas likewise "get the hell outta the Midwest". Nicholas overshot California and the entire Pacific Ocean, landing in Japan, where he lived on and off for five years collectively. During that time, he achieved fluency in Japanese thanks to sage advice from a different friend, who had previously lived in Japan and who insisted, "Don't hang out with other foreigners."

In the US and Japan, Nicholas worked full-time as a systems administrator, and during his mid-twenties he spent several years traveling the world competing as a nationally ranked video game tournament player, but he ultimately gave up the hobby in pursuit of other interests, such as piano composition and photography.

During his late twenties, he toiled over the inverse correlation of his steadily increasing net worth and his steadily decreasing net happiness, and it became obvious that neither spending forty hours per week in an office nor the corporate world in general tickled his fancy. So at the age of thirty, he left a successful and promising career in IT to pursue a lifelong passion far less lucrative but far more enjoyable: writing.

He is particularly interested in anthropology, human sexuality, healthy living, sustainability and minimalism, studies of consciousness (waking, dreaming, and altered states), the beneficial uses of psychedelics, and drug policy reform.

He holds a bachelor's degree in Computer Science, as well as a minor in Mathematics, both of which are now collecting dust. He happily resides in a tiny apartment on the island of Oahu.

You can follow Nicholas at:

facebook.com/WordsByFloyd
twitter.com/words_by_floyd
youtube.com/WordsByFloyd

and on:

nicholasfloyd.com

www.ingramcontent.com/pod-product-compliance
Lightning Source LLC
Chambersburg PA
CBHW051823040426
42447CB00006B/348

9780996173209